W9-DDB-853

Evaluation for Improvement:
A Seven-Step Empowerment Evaluation Approach
For Violence Prevention Organizations
is a publication of the
National Center for Injury Prevention and Control,
Centers for Disease Control and Prevention.

Centers for Disease Control and Prevention
Thomas R. Frieden, MD, MPH, Director

National Center for Injury Prevention and Control
Louise Galaska, MPA, Acting Director

Division of Violence Prevention
W. Rodney Hammond, PhD, Director

Authors
Pamela J. Cox, PhD
Dana Keener, PhD
Tiffanee L. Woodard, MFT
Abraham H. Wandersman, PhD

Editor
Carole A. Craft

Suggested citation:
Cox PJ, Keener D, Woodard T, Wandersman A. *Evaluation for Improvement: A Seven Step Empowerment Evaluation Approach for Violence Prevention Organizations.* Atlanta (GA): Centers for Disease Control and Prevention; 2009.

Acknowledgements

Grantees of the Centers for Disease Control and Prevention's (CDC) Domestic Violence Prevention Enhancements and Leadership Through Alliances (DELTA) Program and the Enhancing and Making Programs and Outcomes Work to End Rape (EMPOWER) Program were instrumental in the development of this publication. All DELTA and EMPOWER Program grantees used an early draft of this manual to hire empowerment evaluators. The experiences, lessons, and insights from their hiring processes are shared throughout this manual.

DELTA Program Grantees

- Alaska Network on Domestic Violence and Sexual Assault
- California Partnership to End Domestic Violence
- Delaware Coalition Against Domestic Violence
- Florida Coalition Against Domestic Violence
- Kansas Coalition Against Sexual and Domestic Violence
- Michigan Coalition Against Domestic and Sexual Violence
- Montana Coalition Against Domestic and Sexual Violence
- North Carolina Coalition Against Domestic Violence
- North Dakota Council on Abused Women's Services/ Coalition Against Sexual Assault
- New York State Coalition Against Domestic Violence
- Ohio Domestic Violence Network
- Rhode Island Coalition Against Domestic Violence
- Virginia Sexual and Domestic Violence Action Alliance
- Wisconsin Coalition Against Domestic Violence

EMPOWER Program Grantees

- Colorado Department of Public Health and Environment
- Kentucky Department for Health and Family Services
- Massachusetts Department of Public Health
- New Jersey Department of Community Affairs
- North Carolina Department of Health and Human Services
- North Dakota Department of Health

Acknowledgements

The following individuals provided substantial input and feedback on earlier drafts of this manual:

Christopher Allen
University of South Carolina

Sandra Cashman
Centers for Disease Control and Prevention

Lorien Castelle
New York State Coalition Against Domestic Violence

Anne Ciemnecki
Mathematica Policy Research , Inc.

Rebecca Cline
Ohio Domestic Violence Network

Jennifer Duffy
University of South Carolina

David Fetterman
Stanford University

Catherine Guerrero
Colorado Department of Public Health and Environment

Wayne Harding
Northeast Center for the
Advancement of Prevention Technology

Jo Ann Harris
North Carolina Coalition Against Domestic Violence

Becca Horwitz
University of South Carolina

Karen Lane
Montana Coalition Against Domestic and
Sexual Violence

Karen Lang
Centers for Disease Control and Prevention

Nicola Miller
Hawaii Department of Health

Janelle Moos
North Dakota Council on Abused Women's Services/Coalition
Against Sexual Assault

Susan Ramspacher
Wisconsin Coalition Against Domestic Violence

Betsy Randall-David
Center for Creative Education

Marilyn Ray
Finger Lakes Law & Social Policy Center, Inc.

Emily Rothman
Boston University School of Public Health

Janice Yost
The Health Foundation of Central Massachusetts, Inc.

Table of Contents

List of Tables

List of Worksheets

Acronyms Used in This Manual

CDC	Centers for Disease Control and Prevention
DELTA	Domestic Violence Prevention Enhancements and Leadership Through Alliances
EMPOWER	Enhancing and Making Programs and Outcomes Work to End Rape
IPV	Intimate Partner Violence
RFP	Request for Proposals
SV	Sexual Violence

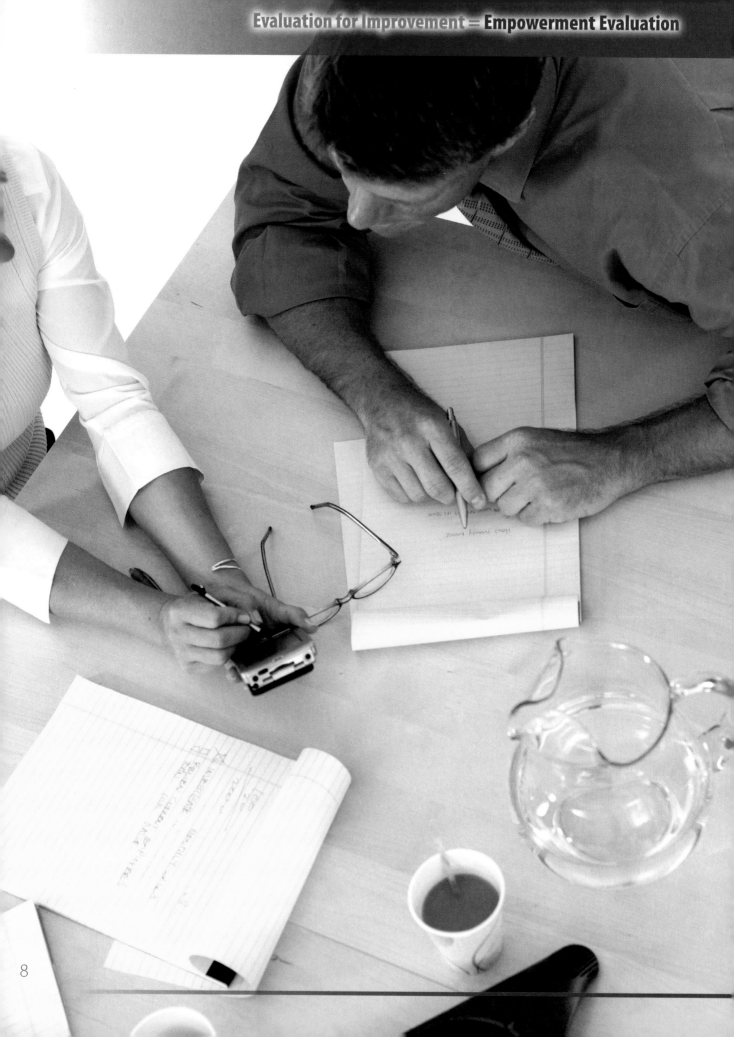

Introduction

Any organization working to prevent violence—whether **sexual violence,**[1] **intimate partner violence, youth violence, suicide,** or **child maltreatment**—wants to know if what it is doing is making a difference. Are **protective factors** against violence increasing? Are **risk factors** for violence decreasing? Are rates of violence decreasing over time? Are there fewer perpetrators and fewer victims than there were in the past? Are communities, families, and individuals healthier and safer now than they were before?

Evaluation can help violence prevention **organizations** answer these and other questions and provide opportunities for these organizations to improve their **strategies**[2] so they are more likely to prevent violence. For this reason, evaluation is becoming a more common practice within organizations, and more funders are requiring grant recipients to evaluate their strategies.

CDC defines **evaluation** as "the systematic collection of information about the activities, characteristics, and outcomes of strategies (i.e., programs) to make judgments about the strategy, improve strategy effectiveness, and/or inform decisions about future strategy development" (based on Michael Patton's definition as cited in U.S. Department of Health and Human Services [U.S. DHHS], 2005, p. 1). What differentiates evaluation from other organizational methods used to assess how strategies are making a difference is a focus on assessing the merit, worth, and significance of a strategy through the systematic collection of information (CDC, 1999). Evaluation can help organizations reduce uncertainties, improve a strategy's ability to achieve its stated goals and outcomes, and make decisions regarding such things as resource allocation (University of Texas – Houston Health Science Center, 1998). For these reasons, evaluation processes and findings can be viewed as complementing, rather than competing with, an organization's regular management processes, including budgeting and strategic planning.

However, evaluation is not always sufficiently well-integrated into the day-to-day management of most organizations. Many reasons account for this. One reason is the concern that evaluation may take time and resources away from strategy implementation. Another reason is that evaluation has traditionally not been structured in a manner that facilitated its integration into the day-to-day operations of an organization. Specifically, organizations have traditionally hired an independent evaluator to conduct an evaluation of their strategies for them (Rossi, Freeman & Lipsey, 1999). These evaluators often worked hard to understand

stakeholders' needs and concerns and develop an evaluation plan to address these concerns and help improve the strategy. The evaluators then submitted an evaluation report to the organization at the conclusion of the evaluation. This report may or may not have been used by the organization to improve its strategies and integrate evaluation into the day-to-day management of the organization. Finally, organizations are often reluctant to pursue evaluation out of concerns that funders may use negative evaluation findings to justify funding reductions.

These concerns and experiences with independent evaluation led to the development of **participatory evaluation** approaches as a way to promote an organization's use of evaluation for the improvement of its strategies. Although there are many participatory evaluation approaches, **empowerment evaluation** places an explicit emphasis on building the evaluation capacity of individuals and organizations so that evaluation is integrated into the organization's day-to-day management processes. Through empowerment evaluation, both **individual and organizational evaluation capacity** are increased through a "learn-by-doing" process, whereby organizations and their staff evaluate their own strategies. Specifically, organizations hire an evaluator to work with them in conducting an evaluation of their strategies. Rather than evaluating an organization's strategies and presenting an evaluation "report card," empowerment evaluators coach individuals and organizations through an evaluation of their own strategy(ies) by providing them with the knowledge, skills, and resources they need to conduct just such an evaluation.

As a result of the empowerment evaluation process, organizational and individual evaluation capacity are improved and a strategy's ability to achieve its stated goals and outcomes is also improved. It is hoped that through empowerment evaluation, evaluation will be established as an essential practice within violence prevention organizations, thereby making our efforts more effective and efficient in saving people from experiencing intimate partner violence, sexual violence, child maltreatment, youth violence, and suicide.

---

[1] All terms in **bold** are defined in the glossary.

[2] The term strategy, rather than **program**, is used in this manual to describe violence prevention efforts across levels (i.e., individual, relationship, community, and society) of the **social ecological model** and to coincide with the empowerment evaluation principles of evidence-based strategies described on page 14. For more information on violence prevention efforts across levels of the social ecology, access Beginning the Dialogue at http://www.cdc.gov/ncipc/dvp/SVPrevention.pdf.

Purpose and Scope of This Manual

This manual is designed to help violence prevention organizations hire an empowerment evaluator who will assist them in building their evaluation capacity through a learn-by-doing process of evaluating their own strategies. It is for state and local leaders and staff members of organizations, coalitions, government agencies, and/or partnerships working to prevent sexual violence, intimate partner violence, youth violence, suicide, and/or child maltreatment. Some parts of the manual may also be useful to empowerment evaluators who work with these organizations.

The manual discusses seven steps an organization might take to hire an empowerment evaluator:

1. Preparing for the hiring process

2. Writing a job announcement

3. Finding potential empowerment evaluators

4. Assessing the candidates

5. Writing an evaluation contract

6. Building an effective relationship with your evaluator

7. Assessing and sustaining the evaluation

The glossary on page 68 defines key terms found in bold throughout the manual. The appendices provide resources, worksheets, and sample documents to make the process of hiring an empowerment evaluator easier.

Additionally, the manual includes "Field Notes," which document the experiences and lessons from CDC's DELTA and EMPOWER Program grantees in hiring empowerment evaluators. The DELTA and EMPOWER Programs are CDC's intimate partner violence

and sexual violence prevention programs, respectively, that have utilized empowerment evaluators to build evaluation capacity at the state and local levels. In the DELTA Program, fourteen state domestic violence coalitions, which are not-for-profit organizations, hired empowerment evaluators to support their development of a data-driven state level intimate partner violence prevention plan and to build the evaluation capacity of local coalitions that received DELTA funding. Through the learn-by-doing process, these empowerment evaluators supported these local coalitions in evaluating their strategies and their capacity building efforts. In the EMPOWER Program, six state health departments hired empowerment evaluators to support their development of a data-driven state level sexual violence prevention plan. Although the DELTA and EMPOWER Programs focus on intimate partner violence and sexual violence prevention, respectively, their experiences and lessons in hiring an empowerment evaluator may be relevant to organizations addressing other types of violence. Their experiences and lessons illustrate practical application of the steps described in the manual by both not-for-profit and state-level government agencies, thereby offering encouragement and highlighting different ways organizations have negotiated the same step. "Notes from the Literature", which are from the published literature on empowerment evaluation, are also provided.

Hiring an empowerment evaluator is a significant step in establishing an ongoing practice of evaluation within your organization. This manual will help prepare your organization to take that step. However, this manual does not describe in detail how to do empowerment evaluation or any other type of evaluation. Resources for conducting general evaluation and empowerment evaluation are provided in Appendix A on page 73.

---

[3] More information on the DELTA and EMPOWER Programs can be found on CDC's website at: www.cdc.gov/violenceprevention/DELTA and www.cdc.gov/violenceprevention/EMPOWER.

Empowerment Evaluation: An Overview

"Empowerment Evaluation aims to increase the probability of achieving program success by 1) providing program stakeholders with tools for planning, implementation, and self-evaluation of their program, and 2) mainstreaming evaluation as part of the planning and management of the program/organization."

Wandersman et al., 2005, p.28

Empowerment evaluation helps organizations improve their efforts to prevent violence by building their capacity to do evaluation and to use evaluation results to improve strategies. Empowerment evaluation is a learn-by-doing process, whereby evaluators train an organization's staff on how to evaluate their own strategies and facilitate the organization's initial evaluation efforts. The long-term goal of empowerment evaluation is for an organization to be able to evaluate its strategies on its own without the assistance of the empowerment evaluator.

The exact structure of the empowerment evaluation training and facilitation process is determined by each organization and their empowerment evaluator. However, the structure generally can be characterized as the empowerment evaluator coaching an organization's staff to:

- Engage stakeholders,
- Describe the strategy,
- Choose an evaluation design,
- Gather credible evidence,
- Write reports that justify their conclusions, and
- Work to ensure that evaluation results are used to improve organizational evaluation capacity and the particular strategy evaluated (CDC, 1999)

Through the empowerment evaluation approach, organizations are able to develop new insights into how their strategies work and what factors support or impede a strategy's ability to achieve positive outcomes (e.g., organizational resources, how staff is trained to implement the strategy). Eventually, organizations are able to conduct their own evaluations without the assistance of the evaluator and integrate evaluation into their day-to-day management practices.

Principles of Empowerment Evaluation

Table 1 lists the 10 principles that define the values and philosophy of empowerment evaluation (Wandersman, et al., 2005). Although some of the principles apply to other types of evaluation as well, the combination of all 10, taken together, makes empowerment evaluation unique. These principles reflect the ideas that individuals are empowered when they are able to work with others, learn decision-making skills, and manage resources and that empowering organizational processes are those that provide opportunities for shared responsibility and leadership (Miller & Campbell, 2006).

The consistent practice of all 10 principles is a goal that organizations are most likely to achieve over time, not something that will immediately occur once an organization decides to use an empowerment evaluation approach. For some organizations, many of the principles will be fully developed at the start of working with an empowerment evaluator. For other organizations, the full development of even a few of these principles will take time. Each organization's current and future demonstration of these principles will be unique. Overall, empowerment evaluators and stakeholders are encouraged to balance the 10 principles in their work and to not let any one single principle dominate their evaluation work.

Organizations should also understand that fidelity to these principles and building individual and organizational evaluation capacity through the empowerment evaluation approach is time consuming. However, the long-term benefit of the empowerment evaluation approach is an organization that is able to continuously improve its strategies and organizational processes without the need of an independent evaluation consultant. Organizations that currently need a more expeditious evaluation of their strategies than empowerment evaluation provides should consider retaining the services of and independent evaluator who can evaluate their strategies for them. (see Harding, 2000).

More information on how to determine if empowerment evaluation is appropriate for your organization is provided in the Step 1: Preparing for the Hiring Process, which starts on page 23.

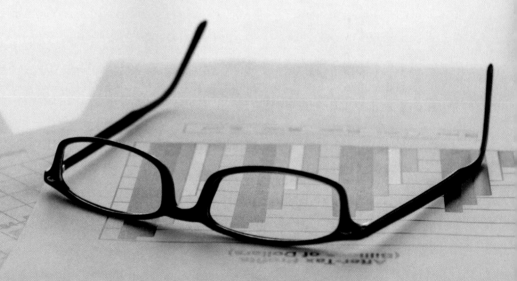

Table 1. Empowerment Evaluation Principles[4]

Principle	Role of the Violence Prevention Organization
Community ownership	Empowerment evaluation places the primary responsibility and ownership for building the organization's evaluation capacity and evaluating the organization's strategies with the organization and not the empowerment evaluator. An empowerment evaluator is just one voice among many. The empowerment evaluator initially provides expertise, coaching, training, tools, and technical assistance to the organization as it evaluates one or more of its strategies and builds its evaluation capacity. Eventually, organizational stakeholders have the capacity to conduct their own evaluations.
Inclusion	Empowerment evaluation involves the representation and participation of key stakeholders.
Democratic participation	Empowerment evaluation is a highly collaborative process. Stakeholders are given the opportunity to voice questions, concerns, and values throughout the evaluation process. Every stakeholder's voice is to be heard and valued equally.
Community knowledge	Empowerment evaluation values and promotes the knowledge present within violence prevention organizations and the communities within which they work. Organizational and community stakeholders, not evaluators, are considered to be in the best position to understand the community's problems and to generate solutions to those problems.
Evidence-based strategies	Empowerment evaluation promotes the use of strategies with high-quality (i.e., **research**) evidence of their **effectiveness** so that organizations can use their resources to select, implement, and evaluate strategies that have a high likelihood of preventing violence. Evidence-based strategies are often complemented by community knowledge to ensure that a strategy is compatible with the community context.
Accountability	Empowerment evaluation provides data that can be used to determine whether a strategy has achieved its goals. Negative results are not punished; rather, they are used to inform changes in a strategy or the selection of a new strategy for the purpose of producing better outcomes.
Improvement	Empowerment evaluation helps organizations to improve their strategies so that they are more likely to achieve their stated goals and outcomes through activities such as needs assessments, assessments of the strategy's design, **process evaluation** and **outcome evaluation** (Rossi et al., 1999).
Organizational learning	Empowerment evaluation fosters a culture of learning within organizations. Stakeholders come to view positive and negative evaluation results as valuable information that guides strategy improvement and to believe that every strategy can be improved.
Social justice	Empowerment evaluation increases an organization's evaluation capacity to implement strategies that work to reduce health disparities that affect groups marginalized (Brennan Ramirez, Baker, Metzler, 2008) by discrimination, persecution, prejudice, and intolerance
Capacity building	Empowerment evaluation builds individual and organizational evaluation capacity so that stakeholders are better able to conduct their own evaluations, understand results, and use them to continuously improve their strategies and their organization.

[4] Based on Wandersman, et al. (2005).

Frequently Asked Questions About Empowerment Evaluation[5]

Why was empowerment evaluation developed?

Empowerment evaluation was developed to overcome practitioner concerns that the independent evaluation structure, whereby an organization hires an external evaluator to evaluate the organization's strategies, often impedes the use of evaluation findings for strategy improvement and the building of the organization's evaluation capacity. Specifically, practitioners have been concerned that under an independent evaluation structure, stakeholders are not adequately engaged in the overall evaluation process and evaluation reports are submitted too late (i.e., often after funding ends) to inform strategy and organizational improvement. Empowerment evaluation attempts to reduce or eliminate these concerns by introducing a different type of evaluation structure that has an empowerment evaluator providing training, technical assistance and tools to organizational stakeholders in how to conduct their own evaluations and improve their organization's evaluation capacity.

Who participates in empowerment evaluation?

Empowerment evaluation is an inclusive process. Ideally, representatives from an organization's key stakeholder groups participate in the empowerment evaluation learn-by-doing process. These key stakeholders include funders, organizational leadership and staff, community participants, and evaluators. These stakeholders hold each other accountable for improving the organization's evaluation capacity and the ability of strategies to achieve their stated goals and outcomes. Together these key stakeholders conduct all the key tasks of an evaluation including describing the strategy, choosing an evaluation design, gathering credible information, writing reports justifying their conclusions, and working to ensure that evaluation results are used to improve organizational evaluation capacity and the particular strategy being evaluated (CDC, 1999).

When is empowerment evaluation appropriate?

Empowerment evaluation is most appropriate when an organization would like to build its own evaluation capacity and improve the ability of its strategies to achieve their stated goals and outcomes on an on-going basis. As used within empowerment evaluation, improving the ability of a strategy to achieve its stated goals and outcomes means describing the strategy based on stakeholders' current understanding, evaluating the strategy, and taking that strategy to its next level of ability to meet its stated goals and outcomes based on the evaluation results and the current resources of the organization. In some cases, improvement will necessitate the choosing of a different strategy in order to achieve the stated goals and outcomes. Evaluating the strategy includes activities such as needs assessments, assessing the strategy's design, process evaluation, outcome evaluation or a combination of these activities (Rossi et al., 1999). Any one of these evaluation activities can produce information that can improve a strategy's ability to achieve its stated goals and outcomes. Like other approaches to evaluation, including independent evaluation, the specific evaluation activities to be used during the empowerment evaluation process to evaluate a particular strategy will be dependent upon various factors such as the purpose of the evaluation, the stage of development of the strategy to be evaluated, and the resources available to conduct the evaluation (Rossi et al., 1999).

Ideally, empowerment evaluation begins in the early stages of strategy planning; however, it can also be used for strategies that are already being implemented. Empowerment evaluation is not as appropriate as research utilizing experimental designs when the purpose of an evaluation is to prove a strategy's effectiveness, typically through the use of control and comparison groups.

Where has empowerment evaluation been used?

Empowerment evaluation has been used around the world in health and human service programs, nonprofit organizations, education, business, foundations, faith communities, and government. It has been used to evaluate strategies and initiatives at local, state, and national levels. Empowerment evaluation can be used anywhere there is a desire to build evaluation capacity for the purpose of improving strategies and integrating evaluation into the organization's day-to-day management processes.

How is empowerment evaluation different from independent evaluation?

As noted above, independent evaluations are often structured in a manner whereby an external evaluator conducts an evaluation of an organization's strategy. The appeal of independent evaluation to many stakeholders, especially funders, is its perceived rigor and objectivity. Independent evaluators may be researchers who utilize their own resources or research funding to determine what will be evaluated and how the evaluation will be done (Rossi et al., 1999). In another type of independent evaluation, an organization

[5] Based on Wandersman & Snell-Johns (2005, p. 422).

may hire an evaluator, who may or may not be a researcher, to determine how an evaluation will be done. In this case, the organization has already determined what will be evaluated and leaves it to the independent evaluator to determine how to conduct the evaluation.

Independent evaluators often consult with stakeholders about a strategy's purpose, implementation, and intended outcomes and then decide how the evaluation should be designed and conducted. The conclusion of many independent evaluations is the submission of an evaluation report that states whether or not the strategy achieved its stated goals and outcomes and recommend how to improve the strategy. Independent evaluation does not make building an organization's evaluation capacity a priority.

However, since the early 1980s many evaluators have questioned the appropriateness of independent evaluation models that utilize the rigor and control standards of academic research for the evaluation of strategies implemented in real world settings that are beyond the control of the organization (Cook & Shadish, 1987; Dugan, 1996; Fetterman, 1982, 1994; Mayer, 1996; Rossi & Freeman, 1989). Additionally, many practitioners have questioned the appropriateness of independent evaluation models that are intended to help improve a strategy, yet provide that very information after the strategy has ended, generally when grant funding has ended. Finally, evaluators and practitioners alike have lamented about how often evaluation findings have gone unread and unused.

Empowerment evaluation seeks to make evaluation more useful to organizations by building individual and organizational capacity to conduct evaluations and use evaluation results to improve strategies and organizational evaluation capacity. With empowerment evaluation, organizations can make corrections to improve their strategies based on real time data. Organizations using an empowerment evaluation approach may use many of the same techniques for data collection and analysis that are used by independent evaluators, but they do so in a manner that reflects the 10 principles of empowerment evaluation and focuses on real-time improvement of strategies and the organization implementing those strategies.

Independent evaluation and empowerment evaluation can complement each other. Empowerment evaluation can be helpful in identifying promising strategies that can then be more rigorously tested through independent evaluation or research for their preventative effects (Fetterman, 2001a).

How is empowerment evaluation different from participatory evaluation?

Participatory evaluation includes a growing variety of evaluation approaches whereby evaluators work with stakeholders to determine what is to be evaluated and how the evaluation will be conducted (Cousins & Whitmore, 1998). The extent of this collaboration can vary tremendously along five dimensions: control of decision making, diversity among stakeholders who participate, power relations among participating stakeholders, manageability of evaluation implementation, and depth of participation (Weaver & Cousins, 2004).

Empowerment evaluation is one type of participatory evaluation that places a strong emphasis on stakeholder control of the decision-making process, a diverse group of participating stakeholders, and active engagement by stakeholders (Weaver & Cousins, 2004). Other types of participatory evaluation can emphasize evaluator control of the decision-making process and minimal participation by only a few stakeholders. Empowerment evaluation also emphasizes a democratic and transparent decision-making process that reduces the possibility of imbalances of power among stakeholders. Other types of participatory evaluation may not address imbalances of power among stakeholders at all. Under all forms of participatory evaluation, including empowerment evaluation, the manageability of evaluation implementation may vary greatly from the evaluation of one strategy to another.

Is empowerment evaluation accurate?

All forms of evaluation are vulnerable to inaccuracies due to errors in design and measurement. Empowerment evaluation results can be as accurate as results from any other form of evaluation. Empowerment evaluation adheres to the Program Evaluation Standards as defined by the Joint Committee on Standards for Educational Evaluation (1994). These standards are grouped into four categories: utility, feasibility, propriety, and accuracy. The standards are intended to ensure that the evaluation meets the information needs of stakeholders and that in meeting these information needs the evaluation is viable, pragmatic, and ethical while producing findings that are considered correct (CDC, 1999). As part of the evaluation capacity-building process, empowerment evaluators should provide tools, training, and technical assistance to the organizations they coach on how to meet these standards when evaluating their strategies.

See CDC's (1999) Framework for Program Evaluation, specifically pages 26–30, and Introduction to Program Evaluation for Public Health Programs: A self-study guide (U.S. DHHS, 2005) for more in-depth discussion and examples of these standards.

What methods are used to do empowerment evaluation?

The particular evaluation methods used to evaluate any strategy are mainly determined by factors such as the purpose of the evaluation, the stage of development of the strategy to be evaluated, and the resources available to conduct the evaluation and not whether or not an empowerment evaluation approach is being used. Thus, the evaluation methods used in an empowerment evaluation are often similar to those used in participatory evaluation or independent evaluation.

Are there specific steps that need to be followed in empowerment evaluation?

There are no specific steps that must be followed within empowerment evaluation. However, three models can inform how organizations and their empowerment evaluators work to evaluate strategies and improve an organization's evaluation capacity.

The first model is from CDC's (1999) Framework for Program Evaluation in Public Health. This model contains six steps: engaging stakeholders, describing the strategy, focusing the evaluation design, gathering credible evidence, justifying conclusions, and ensuring that evaluation results are used. The second model is Fetterman's (2001b) 3-step approach to empowerment evaluation: defining the mission, taking stock, and planning for the future. The third model is Getting to Outcomes, a 10-step approach to planning, implementing, evaluating and sustaining strategies (Chinman, Imm & Wandersman, 2004). These ten steps are: conducting a needs and resources assessment; developing goals and outcomes; selecting evidence-based strategies, assessing the strategy's fit, building capacity, finalizing a plan, conducting a process evaluation, conducting an outcome evaluation, implementing continuous quality improvement, and sustaining efforts.

After reviewing these and other models, organizations and their empowerment evaluators can determine if one model alone, several models in combination or another model would be best to meet their needs.

Who is (or can be) an empowerment evaluator?

An empowerment evaluator is any professional evaluator whose work is guided by the purpose and principles of empowerment evaluation. That is, these evaluators are focused on building individual and organizational capacity so that evaluation can be integrated into the organization's day-to-day management processes. There is no official list of empowerment evaluators to choose from, nor is there a formal way to be certified as an empowerment evaluator. Empowerment evaluators should be chosen based on their willingness, commitment, and ability to focus their work on capacity building and not evaluating strategies themselves.

Is empowerment evaluation appropriate for violence prevention organizations?

Any organization must decide for itself whether empowerment evaluation is appropriate to meet its evaluation needs. However, for several reasons, empowerment evaluation may be a particularly good option for violence prevention organizations. For one, few evidence-based strategies are currently available for the prevention of certain types of violence (i.e., intimate partner violence and sexual violence). Therefore, organizations that want to prevent these types of violence often develop new strategies. Empowerment evaluation is an especially good tool for developing these new strategies because of its focus on utilizing information from needs assessments, assessment of the strategy's design, process evaluation and outcome evaluation for strategy improvement. As noted above, results from these empowerment evaluation activities can be helpful in identifying promising strategies that can then be more rigorously tested by independent evaluation or research for their preventative effects (Fetterman, 2001a). Thus, for fields lacking a substantial inventory of evidence-based strategies, empowerment evaluation can aid in the identification of strategies that may suitable for research studies that could lead to their classification as evidence-based strategies. Empowerment evaluation may also be attractive to violence prevention organizations because of its commitment to community knowledge, community ownership, democratic participation, and social justice.

A more detailed process for deciding if empowerment evaluation is right for your organization can be found in Step 1: Preparing for the Hiring Process, which starts on page 23.

Roles in Empowerment Evaluation

In any evaluation, the organization and evaluator have specific roles and responsibilities. Within empowerment evaluation, funders also have specific roles and responsibilities. Tables 2-4 on the following pages describe each of the roles for the organization, the empowerment evaluator, and the funder in relation to the 10 principles of empowerment evaluation. These roles are ideal. At the outset of an empowerment evaluation process, organizations, empowerment evaluators, and funders may demonstrate only certain aspects of the roles described in Tables 2–4. That's OK. The empowerment evaluation process is intended to be just that—a process, whereby organizations, evaluators, and funders build their capacities over time. A more detailed description of these three roles can be found in Fetterman (2005).

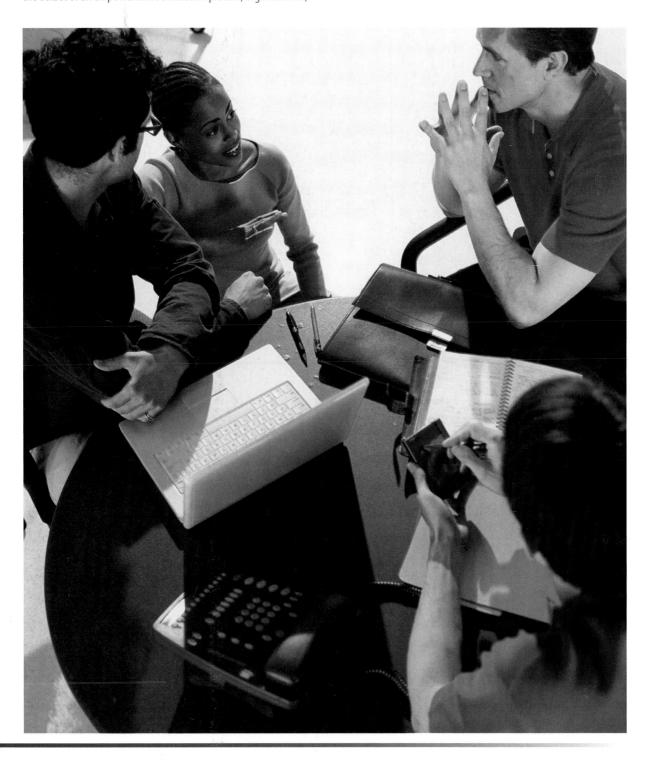

Table 2. Role of the Organization in Empowerment Evaluation[6]

Principle	Role of the Violence Prevention Organization
Community ownership	• Assume responsibility for the oversight and direction of the evaluation capacity–building process and evaluations of specific strategies from the beginning of the contract with your evaluator. • If challenged, defend your organization's ownership of the evaluation capacity–building process, evaluation activities, and any evaluation results
Inclusion	• Invite stakeholders representing the political, religious, and cultural diversity of your organization and community to attend evaluation meetings. • Look for new and diverse partners to help you expand the scope and relevance of your programming and evaluation activities.
Democratic participation	• Commit explicitly to democratic participation as a principle of the evaluation and the evaluation capacity–building process. • Facilitate an environment in which all stakeholders' voices are equally heard and valued. • Develop decision-making processes that are informed by the democratic participation of stakeholders.
Community knowledge	• Use your knowledge of community context, demographics, and conditions to choose prevention goals and strategies and to interpret evaluation findings.
Evidence-based strategies	• Work with your evaluator to identify evidence-based strategies or principles that can lead to your strategies achieving their stated goals and outcomes. • Work with your evaluator to assess whether or not evidence-based strategies need to be adapted to your local community context and conditions. • Work with your evaluator to adapt evidence-based strategies when appropriate.
Accountability	• Evaluate the implementation and outcomes of your strategy. • Identify reasons that actual implementation was different from the plan (process evaluation). • Identify potential reasons that desired outcomes were not achieved (outcome evaluation).
Improvement	• Work closely with your evaluator to improve your organization's evaluation capacity and performance. • Use tools to monitor changes over time in evaluation capacity and strategy outcomes. • Use data to inform decision making for both organizational and strategy improvement.
Organizational learning	• Create an organizational climate that is conducive to institutionalizing and learning from evaluation. • Make decision making as transparent as possible to all stakeholders. • Involve stakeholders in interpreting and evaluating results and in forming recommendations based on the results.
Social justice	• Consider how your organization can extend the potential benefits of your strategy(ies) to all groups within your community, especially those groups who are considered underserved and/or at greater risk for experiencing or perpetrating violence.
Capacity building	• Participate in evaluation training and technical assistance. • Let your evaluator know when you need help or additional coaching in building organizational evaluation capacity or evaluating a particular strategy. • Expect to learn from mistakes.

[6] Adapted from Fetterman (2005).

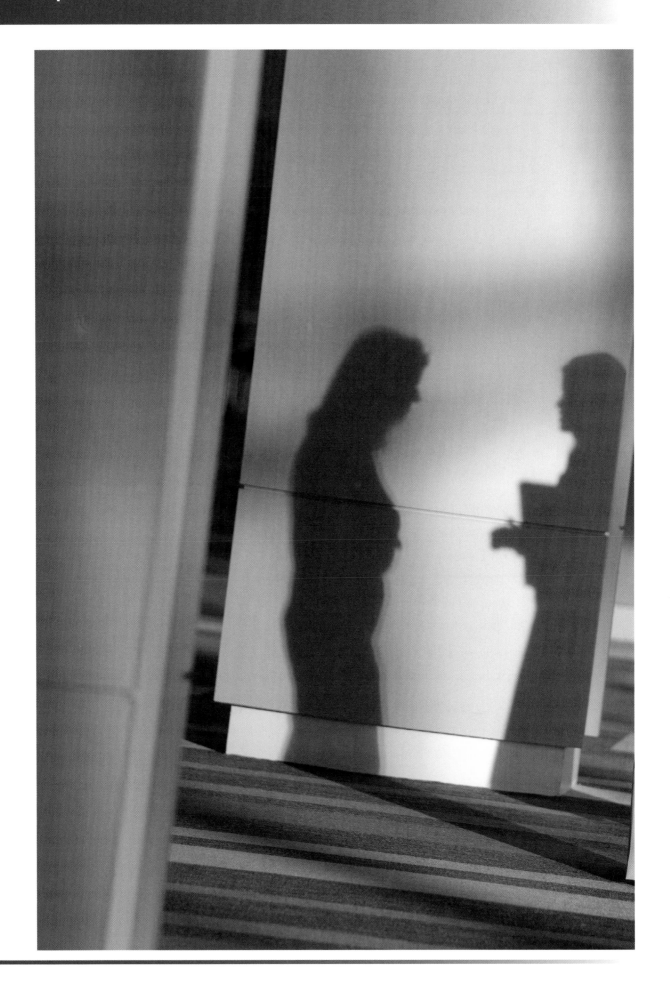

Table 3. Role of the Evaluator in Empowerment Evaluation[7]

Principle	Role of the Evaluator
Community ownership	• Understand that the organization owns the evaluation capacity–building process and the process of evaluating particular strategies. • Serve as a coach rather than a controller of these processes. • Support and encourage organizational staff to take responsibility for the evaluation process, and provide tools and training so that the organization can conduct its own evaluations in the future.
Inclusion	• Know the demographics of the organization and its community. • Ask the organization to invite representatives from key internal and external stakeholder groups to empowerment evaluation meetings and activities, including political and religious leaders and members of different cultural groups in the community served.
Democratic participation	• Facilitate an environment in which all voices are equally heard and valued. • Monitor the level of democratic participation and decision making occurring in the organization and provide feedback.
Community knowledge	• Support the use of organizational and community knowledge in building evaluation capacity and evaluating specific strategies. • Help the organization combine community knowledge with evidence-based strategies.
Evidence-based strategies	• Help identify and promote evidence-based strategies and principles. • Help the organization assess whether or not evidence-based strategies need to be adapted to the local community context and conditions. • Work with stakeholders to adapt evidence-based strategies when appropriate. • Coach organizations to use process and outcome evaluation data to improve their implementation of evidence-based strategies and their organization's capacity-building efforts.
Accountability	• Identify and suggest appropriate tools, measures, and methods to evaluate the results of particular strategies and evaluation capacity–building efforts. • Facilitate an environment in which the organization holds itself accountable for reaching its desired outcomes.
Improvement	• Help the organization focus on improvement, instead of only on problems. • Help the organization use evaluation results for future decision making. • Help the organization internalize the goals, strategies, and desired outcomes of its strategies.
Organizational learning	• Facilitate an environment that values and demonstrates organizational learning. • Help the organization interpret and use data to inform decision making and to make evaluation part of the planning and management of the organization. • Help the organization integrate evaluation in its structures, processes, resources, and programmatic activities.
Social justice	• Help the organization extend the potential benefits of its strategy(ies) to all groups within its community, especially those groups who are considered underserved and/or at greater risk for experiencing or perpetrating violence.
Capacity building	• Provide training and technical assistance to help the organization build its evaluation capacity. • Provide more support early in the evaluation process and gradually reduce support as the evaluation capacity of the organization increases.

[7] Adapted from Fetterman (2005).

Table 4. Role of the Funder in Empowerment Evaluation[8]

Principle	Role of the Funder
Community ownership	• Respect the autonomy of the funded organization. • Encourage organizational and community ownership of the evaluation capacity–building process and the process of evaluating any specific strategies.
Inclusion	• Expect and encourage the evaluation process to be inclusive of all stakeholders. • Provide sufficient financial support for inclusive participation.
Democratic participation	• Support democratic participation with appropriate funding and an appreciation for the additional time required to build evaluation capacity and report results from evaluations of specific strategies.
Community knowledge	• Recognize and validate the use of organizational and community knowledge in planning and evaluation.
Evidence-based strategies	• Expect and encourage the use of evidence-based strategies and principles. • Encourage adaptation of evidence-based strategies to the local community context and conditions when appropriate. • Encourage organizations to use process and outcome evaluation data to improve their implementation of evidence-based strategies.
Accountability	• Work with the organization to measure and report the results of the capacity-building efforts and to use evaluation results to improve strategies. • Support the evaluator in assisting the organization in evaluation of its strategies in a manner consistent with the principles of empowerment evaluation. • Provide sufficient financial support, expertise, and guidance to the evaluation capacity-building effort.
Improvement	• Provide the financial support needed for intensive individual and organizational evaluation capacity building and evaluation. • Participate in problem solving geared towards strategy and organizational improvement. • Encourage the use of an evaluation design that focuses on strategy improvement.
Organizational learning	• Expect organizations to use the evaluation results for future decision making. • Support organizations in sustaining their evaluation capacity–building efforts.
Social justice	• Help the organization extend the potential benefits of its strategy(ies) to all groups within its community, especially those groups who are considered underserved and/or at greater risk for experiencing or perpetrating violence.
Capacity building	• Value and support individual and organizational evaluation capacity building. • Identify and support the use of additional consultants and resources when necessary to build capacity.

[8] Adapted from Fetterman (2005).

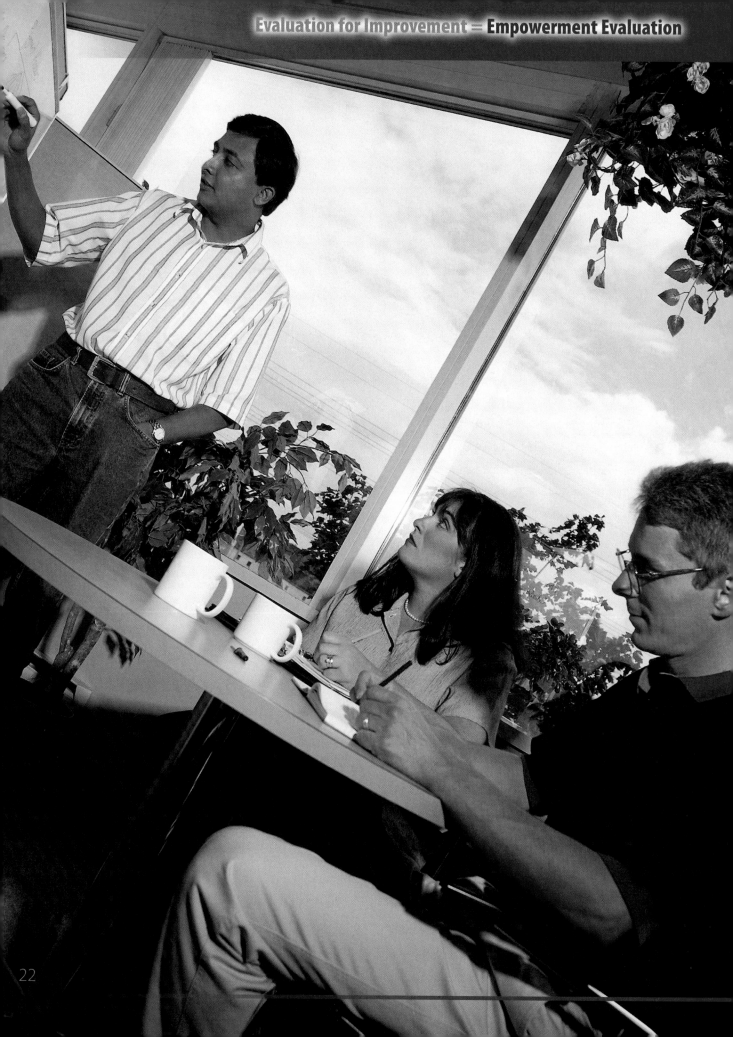

Step 1: Preparing for the Hiring Process

Decide If Empowerment Evaluation Is Right For Your Organization

Empowerment evaluation is particularly well-suited for organizations that want to build their evaluation skills, want their evaluations to be conducted in alignment with their organization's core values (e.g., improvement, community ownership, social justice), and want to institutionalize evaluation within their organization (Miller & Campbell, 2006). What type of outcomes can organizations expect when using an empowerment evaluation approach? They can experience increased use of data for decision making, improvement, and policy work; increases in individual evaluation skills and knowledge; more positive attitudes toward evaluation; and integration of evaluation into the organization's routine activities even after the initial work with an empowerment evaluator ends (Campbell et al., 2004; Miller & Campbell, 2006). Organizations might also see improvements in meeting accountability requirements, collaborating and communicating with stakeholders, protecting funding, engendering a sense of ownership, and sustaining a focus on goals.

When empowerment evaluation is not appropriate

Empowerment evaluation is not appropriate for every organization or every situation. It is inappropriate when:

- The organization is required by a funder to hire an independent evaluator to evaluate one or more of its strategies. In these cases, the funder has decided what will be evaluated and leaves it to the discretion of the independent evaluator to determine how to conduct the evaluation after consulting with stakeholders. This type of evaluation is not empowerment evaluation as the main focus is not on building the organization's capacity to evaluate its strategies. Additionally, the organization's limited ability to control what will be evaluated and how the evaluation will be conducted is not consistent with the empowerment evaluation principle of community ownership.

- The organization is seeking an external evaluator to provide a data-based stamp of approval that their strategies are having a positive impact (Schnoes, Murphy-Berman, & Chambers, 2000). In this case, the organization is not seeking to improve its evaluation capacity through learning by doing, but it does value the rigor and data-driven results produced through an evaluation.

- The organization prefers to use its own subjective standards regarding the success of its strategies, such as the staff's or program director's feeling about the outcomes achieved (Schnoes, Murphy-Berman, & Chambers, 2000). In this case, the organization is not ready for building its evaluation capacity through empowerment evaluation as it does not value the rigor or data-driven results that either an externally conducted or empowerment evaluation can produce.

Is your organization ready for empowerment evaluation?

Although your organization may want to increase stakeholder evaluation skills, conduct its own evaluations that are in alignment with its core values, and institutionalize evaluation (Miller & Campbell, 2006), this desire does not necessarily make the organization or its stakeholders ready to participate in an empowerment evaluation learn-by-doing process. This section provides a general overview of the key issues an organization needs to understand and address to determine if it is ready to use an empowerment evaluation approach. It is important to recognize that no one evaluation approach is appropriate for every organization or for each developmental phase of an organization or a strategy. Just because your organization may not be ready to use an empowerment evaluation approach now does not mean that it won't be in the future. After reviewing the material in this section, your organization will be able to determine if empowerment evaluation is appropriate at this time based on the organization's operating culture and norms.

An organizational culture that supports evaluation capacity building through an empowerment evaluation approach values organizational learning. Such a culture is founded on trust, whereby mistakes are viewed as valuable for the lessons learned not as opportunities for punishment (Preskill & Torres, 1999). Thus, empowerment evaluation is most appropriate for organizations that seek to:

- Increase their organization's talent pool,

- Increase the quality and breadth of information that can help improve strategies,

- Provide a systematic, flexible process for stakeholders,

- Increase the likelihood that evaluation will be undertaken and results will be used,

- Improve communication with audiences by writing evaluation reports in a form appropriate to the needs/interests of different stakeholders (Dugan, 1996).

Empowerment evaluation is not appropriate for organizations that have several of the following operating characteristics and norms (Preskill & Torres, 1999):

- An anti-learning culture,

- Communication channels and systems are underdeveloped or underused to support organizational learning,

- Information is not shared willingly; the organization holds on to a belief that information is power,

- Dialogue and asking questions are not valued,

- Organization members do not generally trust one another,

- There is a fear of making mistakes; risk taking is avoided,

- Independent work is more highly valued than collaborative work,

- Evaluation activity is seen as threatening the status quo,

- Evaluation activity is seen as an "event,"

- Evaluation activity is considered too costly in terms of money, time, and/or personnel resources,

- A general fear of change permeates the organization,

- People are suspicious of any data collection effort.

To help your organization and its stakeholders decide whether empowerment evaluation is right for you and whether your organization is ready to participate in an empowerment evaluation, a deliberative process should be undertaken whereby various issues are considered and debated among various stakeholders. The issues to be addressed are the need for evaluation at this time, current attitudes toward evaluation in general, current attitudes toward empowerment evaluation, and management support for empowerment evaluation. A detailed discussion of each of these topics follows.

Need for evaluation at this time

An organization should first determine what it needs from an evaluation effort at this time. Clarifying this need will help the organization determine which evaluation approach is best.

- Does the organization need to report on the ability of its strategies to achieve their stated goals and outcomes to external

stakeholders, such as funders? If so, a more independent evaluation approach may be the best choice at this time.

- Does the organization need to improve its ability to integrate evaluation into its daily operations and to report its own evaluation findings to stakeholders? If so, an empowerment evaluation approach may be most appropriate.

Current attitudes toward evaluation in general

If stakeholders believe the pros of evaluation are outweighed by the cons at this time, then the introduction of any evaluation approach into an organization may fail because of stakeholders' resistance to evaluation. In these situations, an organization may want to work on increasing stakeholders' positive views of evaluation through training, dialogue, and case studies before taking on any type of evaluation. Once stakeholders see more clearly the benefits of evaluation, the organization should be more receptive and ready to pursue evaluation activities.

Questions to consider in determining your organization's attitude toward evaluation include:

- How do stakeholders feel about the costs, time, resources, and expertise needed to conduct an evaluation?

- Do stakeholders view evaluation as an optional activity with little relevance to strategy implementation or as a key resource to improve their work and the ability of their strategies to achieve their stated goals and outcomes?

- Are stakeholders concerned that an evaluation will not be sensitive to various contextual issues associated with a particular strategy?

- Do stakeholders see evaluation as possibly punitive, exclusionary, or adversarial?

- Are stakeholders motivated to participate in an evaluation?

- In general, is evaluation viewed positively or negatively?

Current attitudes toward empowerment evaluation

Empowerment evaluation requires a great deal of stakeholder time, participation and commitment to ensure the integration of evaluation practices into the organization's day-to-day operations. The following questions can help assess if stakeholders are ready to provide the time, participation, and commitment necessary for empowerment evaluation to succeed in integrating evaluation into an organization's and stakeholders' daily work.

- Are stakeholders prepared to actively participate in various learning activities (e.g., training and technical assistance) to increase their evaluation knowledge, skills, and use? As

Schnoes, Murphy-Berman, and Chambers (2000, p. 59) note, "the empowerment evaluation approach presumes very active participation" and "assumes that clients want and see the need for evaluation of some type."

- Are stakeholders ready to devote time to increasing their evaluation capacity and conducting evaluation activities (e.g., collect data) as part of the learning-by-doing process?

- Are stakeholders prepared for an initial steep learning curve regarding evaluation practice?

- Are stakeholders aware that, as part of the empowerment evaluation process, the evaluator gradually disengages from the evaluation capacity–building process and any evaluations of specific strategies as the stakeholders become more competent

and committed to integrating evaluation into their daily activities (Schnoes, Murphy-Brown & Chambers, 2000)?

- Are stakeholders willing to strive to increase their demonstration of the ideal roles of the organization, empowerment evaluator, and funder (see Tables 2-4 on pages 18–21) as the empowerment evaluation process moves forward?

- What would it mean for the organization and its staff to build its own capacity and to own and control an evaluation of its strategies?

- What type of support from the empowerment evaluator would be best for the organization: coaching, structured guidance, or possibly a combination of the two (Miller & Campbell, 2006)? Table 5 provides more information about these types of support.

Table 5. Empowerment Evaluation: Coaching and Structured Guidance[9]

	Coaching	**Structured Guidance**
Description	Evaluators maintain a question-and-answer relationship with organizational staff and stakeholders. Under this model, the evaluator helps the group decide on the goals, design, and procedures of an evaluation and how the data will be collected, analyzed, and reported. The evaluator helps the group solve problems, provides requested trainings, acts as a sounding board, and poses questions to guide the group in analyzing evaluation findings and determining what they mean for strategy improvement. Evaluators may participate in carrying out evaluation activities as a member of the overall group, not as a lead evaluator.	Evaluators design a set of evaluation steps and how they will be implemented. This design may be done by the evaluator alone or in collaboration with organizational staff and stakeholders. Evaluators may provide evaluation workbooks and worksheets to use in single- or multiple-session trainings for various staff members. Organizational staff members build their evaluation capacity through completing the workbooks and worksheets. Evaluators provide additional training and technical assistance. They sometimes take the lead on analyzing and reporting any data collected.
Situation most often used	Smaller-scale projects	Larger, multi-site projects that make individual coaching difficult
Adherence to empowerment evaluation principles	Closer adherence to the empowerment evaluation principles. Strongest principles: community knowledge, community ownership, and organizational learning. Weakest principles: evidence-based strategies, democracy, social justice, and improvement.	Less adherence to all the empowerment evaluation principles. Strongest principles: accountability, community knowledge, and organizational learning. Weakest principles: democracy, social justice, community ownership, and evidence-based strategies.

[9] Based on Miller & Campbell, 2006.

Management support for empowerment evaluation

Management support and leadership are crucial if the empowerment evaluation approach is to be successful at building both organizational and individual evaluation capacity. The following questions will help your organization determine if management is ready to support and lead the empowerment evaluation process within your organization:

- Is management ready to develop or provide structures, processes, and resources needed for empowerment evaluation to be successful? If so, how?

- Is management ready to ensure that staff's current responsibilities are restructured to allow time for evaluation activities and to communicate that evaluation is not an add-on or optional activity, but one that is integral to the organization's operations?

- Is the organization ready to take a long-term perspective of 5 or more years to build evaluation capacity within the organization (Preskill & Torres, 1999)?

- Does the organization's culture emphasize organizational learning? Is there an organizational norm of trust and courage that supports learning through risk taking (Preskill & Torres, 1999)? Are mistakes viewed as opportunities for learning?

- Is organizational learning supported through democratic processes such as dialogue; reflection; asking questions; and clarifying values, beliefs, assumptions, and knowledge through dialogue and reflection (Preskill & Torres, 1999)?

- Is the organization's leadership willing to integrate evaluation into their daily activities (Preskill & Torres, 1999)? How do they plan to model this?

- Is the organization ready to integrate evaluation into its ongoing operating practices rather than conducting discrete evaluations of specific strategies (Preskill & Torress, 1999)?

- Is management aware of the organizational and community resources available for use in an empowerment evaluation approach? See Worksheet 1: Resources for Empowerment Evaluation in Appendix B on page 76 for additional guidance in this area.

The purpose of these discussions is to identify concerns about evaluation in general, weigh the pros and cons of using the empowerment evaluation approach, and anticipate and address stakeholder questions and concerns about the approach. In some ways, these discussions will be your organization's first opportunity to foster community ownership of your evaluation process, regardless of the approach you choose. At the end of these discussions, your organization will hopefully have a clear understanding of what empowerment evaluation is, what would be required to build your evaluation capacity using this approach, what barriers and facilitators you face, what methods and approaches could be used to minimize barriers and maximize facilitators, and, ultimately, whether or not empowerment evaluation is right for your organization at this time.

At a minimum, these discussions should involve members of the board of directors, management, funders, and staff members who would be affected by the use of an empowerment evaluation approach. Consider having community stakeholders participate as appropriate. As part of these discussions, you may want to invite a speaker who is knowledgeable about empowerment evaluation to do a presentation followed by a question-and-answer session.

Ultimately, the board of directors and/or management must decide what type of an evaluation approach will be used within your organization and whether empowerment evaluation will meet that purpose.

Stakeholders may find it helpful to review the following articles and chapters when assessing if empowerment evaluation is the right approach for your organization at this time:

Campbell, R., Dorey, H., Naegeli, M., Grubstein, L. K., Bennett, K. K., Bonter, F., et al. (2004). An empowerment evaluation model for sexual assault programs: Empirical evidence of effectiveness. *American Journal of Community Psychology, 34*, 251–262.

Livet, M., & Wandersman, A. (2005). Organizational functioning: Facilitating effective interventions and increasing the odds of programming success. In D. M. Fetterman & A. Wandersman (Eds.), *Empowerment Evaluation Principles in Practice* (pp. 123–154). New York: Guilford Press.

Schnoes, C. J., Murphy-Berman, V., & Chambers, J. M. (2000). Empowerment evaluation applied: Experiences, analysis, and recommendations from a case study. *American Journal of Evaluation, 21*(1), 53–64.

Develop a Hiring Plan and Track Your Progress

Once you've decided that your organization will participate in an empowerment evaluation process, you'll need to develop a plan for hiring an evaluator. The remaining sections of this manual are organized around seven steps associated with hiring an empowerment evaluator—each of which may require the completion of several tasks. Both the steps and their associated tasks, outlined in Table 6, can be used to guide the development of a hiring plan; they may also be adapted to better fit your organization's needs.

Table 6. Steps and Tasks in Hiring an Empowerment Evaluator

Step	Tasks
1. Preparing for the hiring process	• Form a hiring committee
2. Writing a job announcement	• Write a job announcement
3. Finding potential empowerment evaluators	• Post job announcement • Identify and contact potential candidates
4. Assessing the candidates	• Review resumes and select candidates for interviews • Interview top candidates • Request and review work samples from top candidates • Conduct a meet and greet of top candidates • Check references of top candidates • Select candidate and make a job offer
5. Writing an evaluation contract	• Develop and sign an evaluation contract with selected empowerment evaluator
6. Building an effective relationship with your evaluator	• Establish an empowerment evaluation team • Exchange information • Establish a communication schedule • Review contract regarding performance issues
7. Assessing and sustaining the evaluation	• Make sure you are really doing empowerment evaluation • Continue the evaluation process after the evaluation contract ends

Form a hiring committee

To foster the principles of empowerment evaluation—particularly community ownership, inclusiveness, and accountability—form a hiring committee (also known as a search committee) that includes members of your organization who have a role and investment in building your organization's evaluation capacity and perhaps in the evaluation of a particular strategy. Worksheet 2: Hiring Committee Checklist in Appendix B on page 78 can help you with this task.

The hiring committee should include someone in leadership within your organization, such as your executive director or program managers, along with the person(s) who will directly supervise the evaluator's work. You should also include the person who is most directly responsible for any initial strategies to be evaluated. You might want to include a front-line staff person who is involved in the direct implementation of the strategy. If your empowerment evaluator will be interacting with members of other organizations

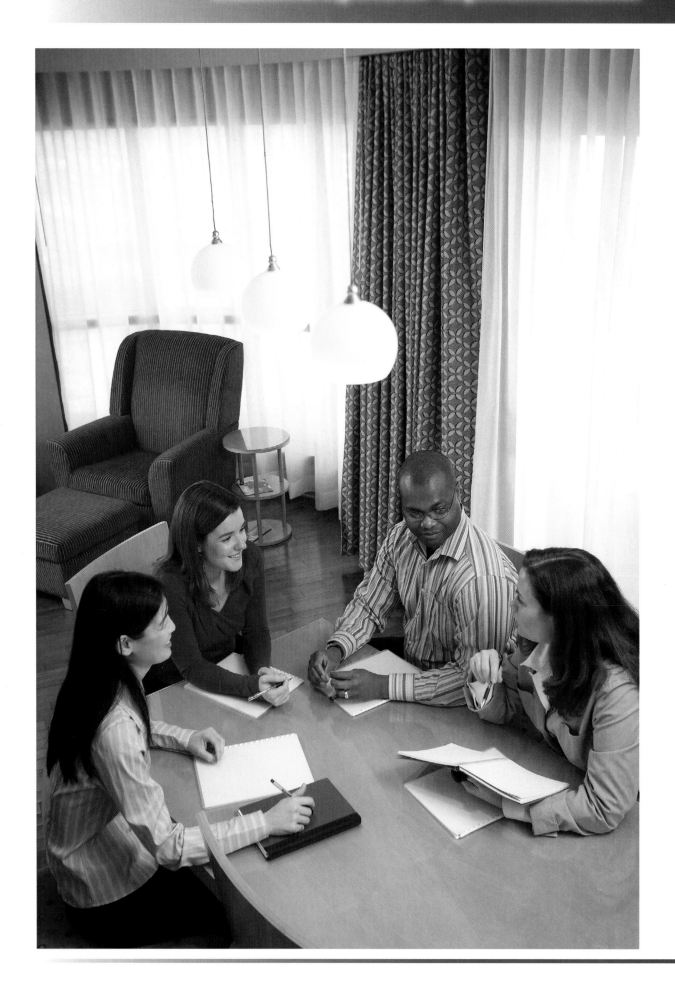

as part of a partnership, it is a good idea to include a representative from those organizations on your hiring committee.

You may also want to include someone with knowledge of various types of evaluation (i.e., independent, participatory and empowerment) and experience in conducting evaluations. If you do not have someone on your staff with such experience, you could invite an evaluator who is familiar with various types of evaluation and who does not wish to apply for the position to be on your hiring committee. Having such a member can be a tremendous asset when you are assessing applicants' qualifications.

Although it is good to be inclusive, your hiring committee needs to be a manageable size, about five to seven people. You can include others in the hiring process without adding them to the hiring committee. For example, once you have narrowed your search to two or three candidates, you could invite staff and other stakeholders to an informal "meet and greet" reception for each candidate. Those who attended the reception can e-mail their comments about each candidate to the hiring committee for consideration in the final selection process.

After your hiring committee is formed, each member should sign a confidentiality statement to protect the privacy of your applicants. A sample confidentiality statement has been provided in Appendix C on page 89.

You'll also want to recap for the committee what empowerment evaluation is, why it is important to this organization, what resources the organization will be able to devote to the empowerment evaluation process (see Worksheet 1 in Appendix B), and the key themes identified in the organization's earlier

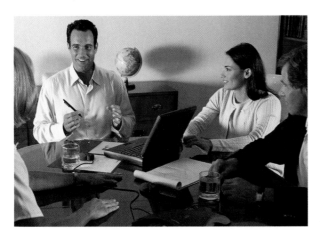

discussions regarding the use of empowerment evaluation. Reviewing this information will ensure that everyone on the hiring committee understands why the organization is looking for an empowerment evaluator and what evaluator qualities will work well with your organization.

Note from the Field

"Each member of the hiring committee represented a programmatic and/or geographic area within the state that the evaluator would be responsible for coaching. For example, one member of the hiring committee represented a rural program and another member was the director of a domestic violence/rape crisis program in a mid-sized community. It was important that each of them participate in the hiring process to ensure that we would hire an evaluator that would be able to work effectively in both communities."

Track your progress

To ensure your hiring process moves along smoothly, develop a plan and method for tracking your progress. Worksheet 3: Tracking Progress for Hiring an Empowerment Evaluator in Appendix B on page 79 can help. This manual does not suggest a timeframe for each step because many variables and factors can affect the time it takes to work through the hiring process. Be realistic about target dates, and be sure to build in extra time around holidays and your organization's busy times. As the hiring process progresses, the hiring committee may adjust target dates because of unforeseen circumstances or tasks that took longer than expected. The important thing is to complete each task in a thoughtful and deliberate manner.

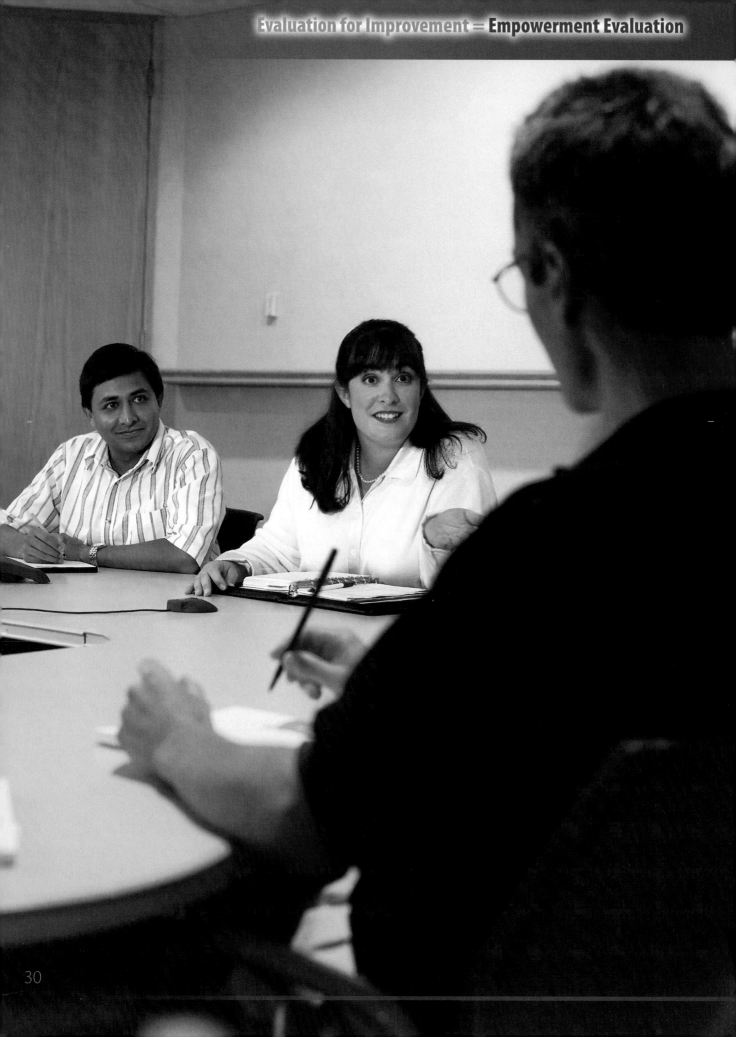

Step 2: Writing a Job Announcement

A job announcement for an empowerment evaluator is the primary way to communicate the qualifications you desire and the deliverables you expect. It may be similar to other job announcements your organization has created.

The job announcement should be specific and clear so potential applicants can determine if they are qualified for the position and if the position is of interest to them. A good job announcement will increase the likelihood that you will find appropriate applicants and will reduce the time you spend reviewing applications from inappropriate candidates. It should be brief (not more than 1–2 pages) and easy to read. Use bold and italics to highlight words that you want to stand out.

Note from the Field

"At the beginning of the hiring process, the most important lesson that we learned was to be flexible with the process and identify priorities (experience with domestic/sexual violence and evaluation). Therefore, what is put into the job announcement has to be well thought out and agreed upon by the hiring committee, with clearly stated non-negotiables."

Common components of a job announcement include the following:

- Name and description of hiring organization
- Title of position
- Type of position (e.g., part-time, contractual)
- Length of project or contract
- Summary of position
- Job responsibilities and deliverables
- Minimum and preferred qualifications
- Available compensation
- Application instructions and deadline

A sample job announcement is included in Appendix D on page 90.

Some organizations may announce their position through a request for proposal (RFP). An RFP includes many of the same elements as a job announcement; the main difference is that an RFP requires that the applicant submit a proposal with a detailed plan of work. A sample RFP is available in Appendix E on page 91.

Define the Type of Position

Your organization's empowerment evaluation needs can be filled by offering a staff position or a contract position. A contract position is the most popular choice because it is flexible and usually costs less than hiring a staff member. Hiring an evaluator as a full-time or part-time employee, although typically more costly, has the potential to significantly increase an organization's evaluation capacity.

If you offer a contract position, your job announcement should include an estimate of the time the position will require, such as the number of hours or days per week or per month. It can be difficult to estimate the amount of time required for the position, especially if this is the first time you have worked with a contract evaluator. For this reason, you may want to add a clause in the job description that the estimated time involved is subject to change.

If you are uncertain about whether to offer a staff position or a contract position, you can wait until you have reviewed your applicant pool to decide which arrangement is most feasible.

Define Responsibilities and Deliverables

The responsibilities of the position define what you expect your empowerment evaluator to do. Deliverables are what you expect your empowerment evaluator to do and produce, such as developing a training manual and then providing a training with follow-up technical assistance as stakeholders apply the training materials to the evaluation of a specific strategy.

Notes from the Field

"We initially decided to have the empowerment evaluator as a staff position, so we didn't interview folks that applied as a contract position. Then we decided to contract the position. If we could do it all over again, we would make our decision regarding whether this would be a contract or staff position after we interviewed all qualified candidates."

"Our evaluator is employed by our organization. We made the decision to make this a staff position after our State Department of Health agreed to allow us to apply some of our annual award to the salary and benefits of this position as well. This allowed us to maintain our commitment to equity in our work on behalf of both sexual and domestic violence…and to build our capacity to sustain this work in the future."

Because empowerment evaluation is collaborative, you may expect that your evaluator will contribute to the production of certain deliverables (e.g., evaluation reports), but may be solely responsible for others (e.g., providing written recommendations on how to institutionalize evaluation within the organization or a group training on process evaluation that includes a PowerPoint presentation and manual).

The job responsibilities and deliverables should be based on the needs of your organization, which you defined while deciding whether empowerment evaluation is right for your organization, and on any evaluation requirements of specific strategies as defined by your funder(s). Table 7 provides a list of common job responsibilities of an empowerment evaluator. These responsibilities may or may not be appropriate for your organization. The list is provided to help you think about what your organization needs from your empowerment evaluator. You can record your needs on Worksheet 4: Defining Job Responsibilities and Deliverables, found in Appendix B on page 80.

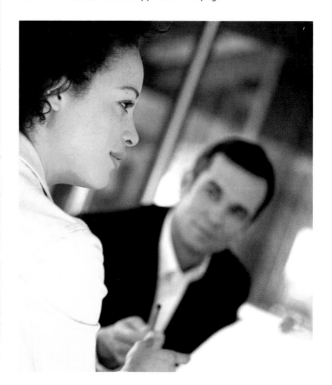

Table 7. Common Job Responsibilities and Deliverables of an Empowerment Evaluator

Adhere to the principles of empowerment evaluation

Empowerment evaluators should know the 10 empowerment evaluation principles and constantly assess whether or not they are living up to these principles in their work with a particular organization. For instance, it is quite common for an empowerment evaluator to question if he or she is owning/controlling the evaluation capacity-building process and the evaluation of any specific strategies in a manner that weakens the principles of community ownership and capacity building. It is also quite common for members of the organization to develop their ownership of the evaluation process over time; that is, substantial community ownership by the organization and its staff may not happen until they gain a better understanding of evaluation concepts, practices, and processes (Keener , Snell-Johns, Livet, & Wandersman, 2005).

Assess the evaluation needs and resources of staff and the organization

Empowerment evaluators should meet with organizational staff and other stakeholders to learn about the organization's history, management structure, core values and hierarchy, funding resources, strategies, clients and constituents, community partnerships, and past and current evaluation activities (Campbell et al., 2004). Empowerment evaluators can then provide a written report that describes the organization's needs and resources and provides recommendations on how to increase the evaluation capacity of the organization and its staff.

Conduct or facilitate training and technical assistance to develop individual and organizational evaluation capacity

Empowerment evaluators are responsible for using adult learning principles, collaboration, and facilitation/coaching techniques to increase individual and organizational evaluation capacity. Preskill and Torres (1999) emphasize the use of four learning processes when building evaluation capacity: dialogue; reflection; asking questions; and identifying/clarifying values, beliefs, assumptions, and knowledge. It is unacceptable for an empowerment evaluator to simply provide PowerPoint presentations that do not encourage questions, dialogue, and real application to the organization's current issues.

Empowerment evaluators provide training and technical assistance on such topics as how to:

- Engage stakeholders
- Describe the strategy
- Choose an evaluation design
- Gather credible information
- Write reports that justify conclusions
- Work to ensure that evaluation results are used to improve organizational evaluation capacity and the particular strategy evaluated (CDC, 1999).

Training and technical assistance should include skills-based activities, not just lecture. Empowerment evaluators can review reports required by funders from an evaluation perspective so as to better report evaluation findings to funders. Empowerment evaluators can assess the feasibility and outcomes of logic models developed by an organization and help an organization understand the utility of required reports beyond just satisfying a funder's reporting requirements.

Under a structured guidance empowerment evaluation, the evaluator may develop a training curriculum. Any training materials created should be easy to read, be adaptable for multiple purposes, be usable by participants who are unable to attend a training, and provide real-life examples of violence prevention strategies (Campbell et al., 2004). Manuals and guides may be used to support the training curriculum. Topics may include data analysis/use as well as resources for evaluation, such as data analysis software.

Continued

Table 7. Common Job Responsibilities and Deliverables of an Empowerment Evaluator (Continued)

Promote critical thinking and consensus building

Empowerment evaluators also have a key role in promoting critical thinking and building consensus among stakeholders about what is learned from the evaluation and how findings are applied to strategy and organizational improvement. As various stakeholders may have different priorities, evaluators are charged with using the 10 empowerment evaluation principles as a framework through which to facilitate group discussions and reach decisions.

Facilitate and assist in the development of an evaluation plan for specific strategies that takes into consideration each strategy's stage of development and the organization's capacity

Empowerment evaluators do not write the evaluation plan for stakeholders to review. Rather, through training, technical assistance, and facilitation, they enable stakeholders to develop their own plans.

Provide coaching and assistance in collecting, storing, and analyzing data

Empowerment evaluators initially provide hands-on coaching and assistance in collecting, storing, and analyzing data, which tapers off over time as the organization gains capacity in these areas.

Assist in the completion of specific reporting requirements

Empowerment evaluators coach the organization and its staff on how to include evaluation findings in specific reporting requirements. This coaching may be more hands-on early in the process and taper off as both individual and organizational evaluation capacity increase.

Travel to periodic trainings and meetings sponsored by funders

Empowerment evaluators may be required to attend trainings and meetings sponsored by the organization's funders. Empowerment evaluators understand that they do not have the authority to speak for the organization when attending such meetings unless the organization gives them such authority. In these situations, the evaluator is careful to present himself or herself not as the evaluation expert regarding the organization's strategies, but as a coach working to increase the organization's evaluation capacity.

Define Required and Preferred Qualifications for the Position

Your hiring committee should develop a list of qualifications that are necessary and realistic to expect of your empowerment evaluator. The list should be informed by the needs of your organization, as identified in the discussions that led to your decision to hire an empowerment evaluator. At times, the hiring committee may have to use its own judgment to determine what these qualifications are. Every effort should be made to ensure that the qualifications align with the needs and perspectives of the organization.

The size of your expected applicant pool is an important factor when deciding which qualifications to require vs. those that are preferred. If your organization is located in a large metropolitan area, for example, you may be able to set relatively high qualification standards to avoid receiving too many applications. However, if your organization is located in a small, rural area where there may be fewer evaluators to choose from, you may want to set both minimum and preferred qualifications. That way, you can remain open to a wider range of potential candidates while also defining your ideal candidate.

The combination of qualifications is important. None of the qualifications described in this section are meant to stand alone. For example, someone may meet the suggested educational qualifications but not have the evaluation experience, evaluation capacity–building experience, or the facilitation skills you are looking for.

Table 8 suggests qualifications for an empowerment evaluator. After reviewing these qualifications, your hiring committee can use Worksheet 5: Defining Qualifications of the Position (in Appendix B on page 81) to describe those that are most important to your organization. Your hiring committee will also need to determine how it will assess these qualifications. For instance, a potential candidate's facilitation skills will not be easily assessed by reviewing a resume or conducting an interview with the candidate. Your hiring committee may need to get references that can report their observations of a potential candidate's facilitation skills.

Table 8. Suggested Qualifications for an Empowerment Evaluator

	Not qualified/ Not a match	Qualified (Required)	Qualified (Preferred)
Education/training	No graduate degree	Master's degree in public health, psychology, education, or other related field Coursework in evaluation and/or research methods and statistics	Doctoral degree (PhD) in public health, psychology, education, or other related field Coursework in additional relevant subject matter (specified by your organization)
Previous professional experience	No practical experience doing participatory or community-based evaluation (even if highly experienced as a researcher)	At least 2 years of professional experience doing participatory or community-based evaluation with an emphasis on organizational capacity building	At least 4 years of professional experience doing participatory or community-based evaluation with an emphasis on organizational capacity building Has done empowerment evaluation with community-based organizations
Orientation to evaluation	Believes that evaluation is only valid when conducted by a professional evaluator Is unwilling to use an empowerment evaluation approach	Views evaluation as a tool for strategy development and improvement; believes that evaluation can be done by organizational stakeholders when equipped with the skills and tools to do evaluation Is enthusiastic about using an empowerment evaluation approach	Views evaluation as a tool for strategy development and improvement; believes that evaluation can be done by organizational stakeholders when equipped with the skills and tools to do evaluation Experience in participatory or empowerment evaluation approaches
Facilitation skills	Is unable to facilitate a group decision-making process in accordance with the 10 empowerment evaluation principles	Is developing the ability to facilitate a group decision-making process in accordance with the 10 empowerment evaluation principles	Is able to facilitate a group decision-making process in accordance with the 10 empowerment evaluation principles
Communication skills	Poor verbal and written communication skills	Strong verbal and written communication skills	Excellent verbal and written communication skills

Education and training

Professional evaluators, including empowerment evaluators, come from a range of academic fields and educational backgrounds. Qualified evaluators typically hold graduate degrees in public health, psychology, education, or social work. Whatever an evaluator's field, look for completed coursework in research or evaluation methods and statistics.

Individuals with doctoral degrees in one of the areas listed above have typically completed an intensive research requirement that can be good preparation for doing professional evaluation. Although a PhD is certainly desirable, individuals with master's degrees often have the education and skills needed to do evaluation.

There is no formal training program for empowerment evaluation, nor are there special courses taken only by empowerment evaluators. Therefore, although educational background will help you determine who has the basic knowledge to do evaluation of any type, it will not tell you who might be good at coaching an organization in building its evaluation capacity and through the initial evaluation of the organization's strategies. Other qualifications will be more important in making that distinction.

In addition to formal education, some evaluators pursue training opportunities through workshops and institutes, such as the annual meeting of the American Evaluation Association and the annual Summer Evaluation Institute sponsored by the American Evaluation Association and the Centers for Disease Control and Prevention. Some institutes occasionally offer workshops specifically on empowerment evaluation. Although you may not want to limit your search to candidates who have participated in such training opportunities, these experiences suggest that a candidate is making a concerted effort to grow in his or her abilities as an evaluator overall and perhaps as an empowerment evaluator in particular.

Depending on the expected size of your applicant pool, you may also want to consider specific educational background or coursework that informs your organization's prevention efforts. For example, evaluators with public health education and experience are likely to be familiar with primary prevention concepts, evaluation, and working with community-based organizations to achieve positive health outcomes. Evaluators with education and experience in women's studies may be particularly well suited to organizations that want to ensure that the empowerment evaluator has a sufficient understanding of the principle of social justice and that this understanding informs how he or she provides training,

technical assistance, and coaching, especially in the interpretation of evaluation results. Evaluators with a background in school psychology or developmental psychology may be desirable to organizations focused on youth development.

Professional experience

Professional experience in four key areas is highly desirable for an empowerment evaluator:

1. Experience working from a participatory evaluation perspective. One might assume that a viable candidate for empowerment evaluator must have previous experience doing empowerment evaluation. Although this would be ideal, it might not be a realistic expectation in all cases. Empowerment evaluation is still a relatively new approach to evaluation, and while more opportunities to use the approach are emerging all the time, many professional evaluators who appreciate the values of empowerment evaluation may not have had the opportunity to apply the approach. Evaluators who have worked from other participatory evaluation approaches may be very qualified candidates to do empowerment evaluation, if they are willing to adjust their approach to focus more on individual and organizational capacity building. Therefore, your organization may place more emphasis on whether or not a potential candidate's overall approach to evaluation is conducive to empowerment evaluation than on previous experience doing empowerment evaluation specifically. If you have a large applicant pool, you may still have the option of choosing someone with a specific background in empowerment evaluation.

2. Experience working with diverse stakeholders who are not trained evaluators. Your empowerment evaluator will be responsible for building evaluation capacity among your stakeholders and within your organization. Having experience in working with diverse stakeholders who are not trained evaluators may help an empowerment evaluator build a collaborative atmosphere more quickly and increase staff ownership of the evaluation capacity–building process.

3. Experience conducting or facilitating evaluations driven by organizational needs. Candidates for the empowerment evaluator position should have experience in helping organizations do evaluation that is driven by organizational needs, rather than by the evaluator's own interests. Ideally, your empowerment evaluator will have experience with an organization whose culture, resources, and perspective on collaboration with other community partners is similar to yours. This experience will provide a basis for the evaluator to understand what activities to pursue, and how quickly to pursue them, in building your organization's evaluation capacity.

An evaluator who has conducted evaluation activities based only on his or her interests is not a good candidate for your organization's empowerment evaluator.

How much evaluation experience is enough? There is no simple answer to this question, but more experience is usually better than less. In most cases, at least 2 years of evaluation experience is adequate, and 4 or more years of experience is preferable. Evaluation experience consists of work experiences in which the applicant worked independently, or as part of a team, either conducting an evaluation or building organizational evaluation capacity. Look for previous job titles such as "program evaluator," "evaluation specialist," "director of evaluation," and "evaluation consultant."

4. Experience in organizational and individual evaluation capacity building. Because of empowerment evaluation's emphasis on capacity building, candidates for the empowerment evaluator position should ideally have experience in building both individual and organizational evaluation capacity. Individual evaluation capacity–building experience may have come from teaching evaluation courses within a university or other setting. Organizational evaluation capacity–building experience may have come from prior work with organizations that wanted to integrate evaluation into their day-to-day management processes. The main point is to specifically assess how each candidate has worked to build evaluation capacity within individuals and organizations and/ or what their perspective is on how they would do this within your organization.

You may also want to highlight some other types of specialized experience in your job announcement. For example, if your organization is working as part of a community partnership or using a community mobilization approach, you may want an empowerment evaluator who has worked with and evaluated the efforts of community coalitions.

Again, the size of your expected applicant pool will determine whether you list these types of experiences as required or preferred qualifications.

Orientation to evaluation

The most important factor for distinguishing potential empowerment evaluators from other types of evaluators is their orientation to evaluation. At a minimum, you should require that applicants be willing to work with your organization to build its evaluation capacity in a manner that is consistent with the principles of empowerment evaluation, regardless of their previous experience in doing so. It might be helpful to list the principles of empowerment evaluation in your job announcement.

Specifically, candidates for an empowerment evaluator position should view evaluation as an organizational tool for strategy development and improvement. They should also believe that organizational stakeholders can conduct evaluation accurately when they are equipped with the skills and tools they need. In addition, they should believe that evaluation can be useful and relevant to stakeholders, especially when stakeholders own and participate in the evaluation process.

Independent evaluators who are more comfortable doing an evaluation than building individual and organizational evaluation capacity in a learn-by-doing process would probably not be good empowerment evaluators.

Facilitation skills

Empowerment evaluators are charged with building organizational and individual evaluation capacity in a manner consistent with the 10 principles of empowerment evaluation. To balance principles such as social justice, community knowledge, evidence-based strategies, and accountability among a group of stakeholders working to improve a strategy, an empowerment evaluator must have strong facilitation skills. Experience in building consensus and reaching compromise is vital to this position.

Communication and interpersonal skills

Effective communication skills are essential for an empowerment evaluator. An individual in this position should be able to write and speak clearly, using terms that are easy to understand. In addition, he or she should be capable and comfortable in speaking to both small and large groups. The ideal candidate should have experience providing training and technical assistance in a variety of settings, should understand the needs of adult learners, and enjoy being in a coaching role. Your evaluator should have experience forming strong working relationships with a diverse array of organizational stakeholders. Ultimately, you want someone with whom you and your staff feel comfortable—someone who is supportive and non-threatening and can interact with you about evaluation using everyday language.

Other conditions of employment

Your job announcement should also specify any other conditions of employment that are important to your organization. For instance, is it necessary that the evaluator live in the same state or community where your organization is located? Do you need an evaluator who is bilingual or has special language skills? Will travel be required, and how often?

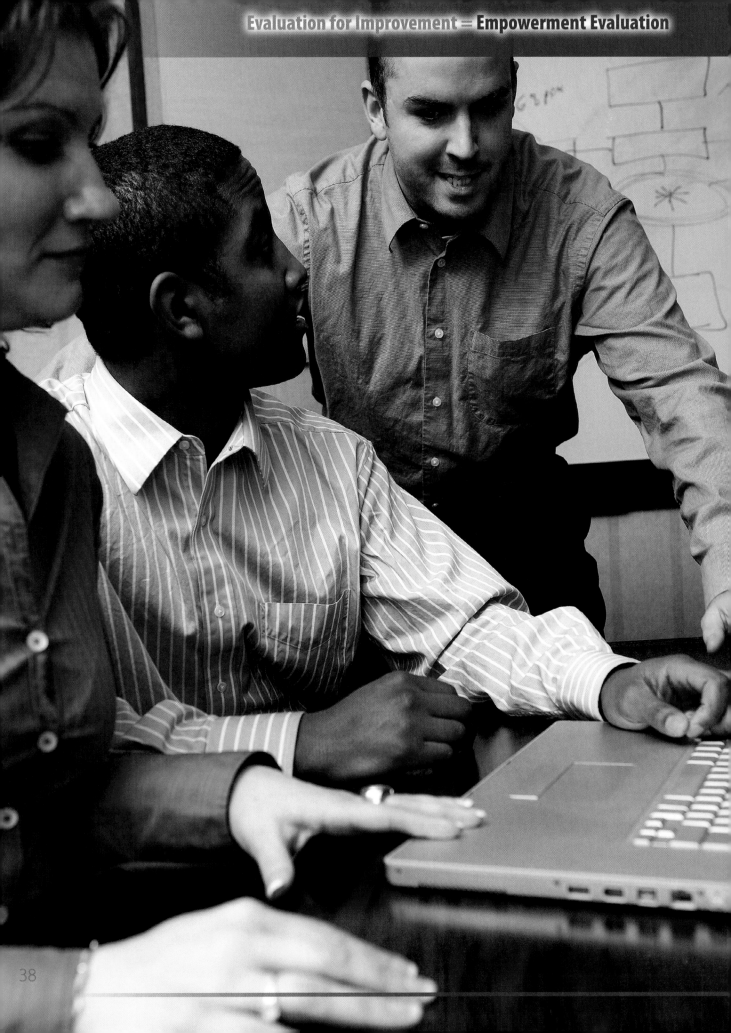

Step 3: Finding Potential Empowerment Evaluators

Know Where to Look for Candidates

Empowerment evaluators, like most other evaluators, typically work in a university or other academic setting, in a research or evaluation consulting firm, or as independent consultants (i.e., they are self-employed and/or have their own small business). In addition, many evaluators have full-time positions in nonprofit organizations and government agencies; unless they are willing to change jobs, however, these individuals are usually not available for other projects. Keep in mind that the setting within which an evaluator works says nothing about his or her inclination or skills to practice empowerment evaluation. That is something you will assess based on the resumes you receive and interviews you conduct with your candidates.

This section presents some of the advantages and disadvantages of working with evaluators from different professional settings, as well as issues associated with working with an evaluation team.

University-based evaluators

University-based evaluators are employed as faculty or may work for a faculty member at colleges or universities.

Advantages of using university-based evaluators:

- Can bring a high level of prestige, scholarship, and expertise to an empowerment evaluation project.

- Can have extensive experience in teaching evaluation due to teaching and dissertation or thesis responsibilities

Disadvantages of using university-based evaluators:

- These evaluators generally have multiple demands on their time, such as teaching, conducting research, writing publications, and possibly consulting with other clients, which may limit their focus on your organization's empowerment evaluation activities.

- When hiring a university-based evaluator, the university typically applies indirect fees, ranging from 25%–50%, in addition to the cost charged by the faculty consultant. The indirect fees are intended to support university overhead expenses (e.g., utilities, building maintenance). More information about how to negotiate indirect costs during the contracting phase will be discussed in Step 5: Writing an Evaluation Contract, which starts on page 55.

University-based evaluators frequently involve graduate students in their projects. This may reduce the cost of hiring a university-based evaluator, and it may allow professors to accept projects that they may not otherwise have the time to do all by themselves. However, be mindful of the fact that graduate students are still learning about evaluation generally, empowerment evaluation specifically, and possibly the subject matter your organization addresses. This learning curve can delay the empowerment evaluation process. Also, a professor and his or her graduate students form an evaluation team, which can present special challenges; these are discussed separately in a following section.

Research/evaluation consulting firms

Research/evaluation consulting firms are usually private, for-profit companies that employ professionals with particular types of expertise in research and evaluation. Consulting firms can range in size from just a few employees to hundreds of employees spread across the country. Some firms may specialize in working with certain types of clients (such as nonprofits or government agencies) or within particular content areas.

Advantages of working with a research/evaluation consulting firm:

- Their sole focus is on serving clients.

- They generally have a sizeable infrastructure of resources and skills from which to draw to support your organization. Rather than depending on one person to carry out all phases of a project, they might have one person who focuses on measurement, another who focuses on analysis, and another who focuses on capacity building.

Disadvantages of working with a research/evaluation consulting firm:

- These firms also have multiple demands on their time due to having multiple clients, which may limit their ability to focus on your organization's empowerment evaluation activities at certain times.

- Often multiple personal will be assigned to a specific project, each with varying degrees of experience with evaluation in general and empowerment evaluation in particular.

- Key personnel on the project may leave the organization or get moved to another project.

- Management of an evaluation team assigned to your organization may require much more time and resources than working with just one staff member. The issues associated with working with an evaluation team are discussed below.

- Consulting firms charge substantial overhead or indirect costs, which are often in the same range as those charged by universities: 25-50% of the direct costs.

Independent evaluation consultants

Independent evaluators are generally professionals who are self-employed and consult with a number of different clients.

Advantage of working with an independent evaluation consultant::

- They have complete control over the work demands they choose to accept, as opposed to being assigned projects by a supervisor at a firm or needing to balance teaching responsibilities at a university.

Disadvantages of working with an independent evaluation consultant:

- The evaluator will likely need to balance the needs of several clients simultaneously.

- Your organization is highly dependent upon the expertise and availability of one person. If your chosen evaluator lacks expertise in a particular area, you may incur additional costs or time delays while the evaluator works to get up to speed in that area. Also, if your chosen evaluator becomes unavailable for some reason (e.g., illness, family emergency, client conflicts), there is no one to act as a back up.

Evaluation teams

Occasionally, independent consultants team up with other independent consultants or a university-based evaluator for larger projects. And, as noted above, you may also encounter a team if you hire an evaluation firm or a university-based evaluator who enlists the assistance of graduate students. If managed well, an evaluation team can afford your organization tremendous benefits, as they can offer access to more resources and expertise. If managed poorly, however, working with such a team can be taxing and leave members of your organization with a negative attitude toward evaluation.

To manage evaluation teams properly, you must establish clear roles and expectations for all team members, including those from your organization. This will help reduce duplication of efforts and minimize delays when staff turnover occurs because everyone will know which responsibilities now need to be transferred to someone else.

When hiring an empowerment evaluation team, set clear expectations and agreements about who will be doing the majority of the day-to-day project management. If it is a graduate student or a junior evaluator at a consulting firm, make sure this person has the desired education, evaluation experience, orientation to evaluation, project management experience, facilitation skills, and communication skills. Additionally, find out how the university-based professional, research/consulting firm, or independent evaluator has managed evaluation teams previously, what they learned from those experiences, how they handle client concerns, and what quality-assurance processes they implement to ensure your organization gets what it needs.

Advertise Your Position

To reach a wide audience of qualified empowerment evaluators, it is not enough to simply post your job announcement or request for proposals (RFP) in the local newspaper. A more proactive approach is needed. Here are some steps you can take to advertise your position to the most appropriate potential candidates.

Listservs

Professional organizations typically use listservs to promote discussions about topics relevant to a particular profession and to share information about available positions within a profession. Some listservs reach a national or even international audience of professionals within a particular field. The most well-known listserv for evaluators in the United States is administered by the American Evaluation Association. In addition, evaluators often subscribe to listservs for other fields that are not exclusively focused on evaluation, such as public health, psychology, prevention research, and education. Table 9 provides a short list of some of the national listservs that are likely to reach current or potential empowerment evaluators. You may want to search for regional, state, or local listservs as well.

Table 9. Listservs for Locating Potential Empowerment Evaluators

Host Organization	Web/Email Address
American Evaluation Association (AEA)	The American Evaluation Association lists many evaluation-associated listservs on their website at www.eval.org/Resources/Listservs.asp. Three evaluation listservs that may be most helpful in identifying empowerment evaluators are: **AEA LIST NAME:** EVALTALK **Topics:** All types of evaluation **Sponsor:** Official list of the American Evaluation Association **Information link:** http://bama.ua.edu/archives/evaltalk.html **For assistance contact:** Kathleen Bolland at kbolland@sw.ua.edu **AEA LIST NAME:** Empowerment Evaluation **Topics:** Collaborative, participatory and empowerment (CPE) evaluation **Sponsor:** CPE Topical Interest Group (TIG) of the American Evaluation Association **Information Link:** http://www.eval.org/TIGs/empower.html **For assistance contact:** David Fetterman at davidf@leland.stanford.edu **LIST NAME:** SCRA **Topics:** Community research and action, information on job postings, grant opportunities, and SCRA events. **Sponsor:** Society of Community Research and Action **Information link:** http://www.apa.org/divisions/div27/elistserves.html **For assistance contact:** scra-lists@prodigy.net
Stanford University Empowerment Evaluation Listserv	empowerment-evaluation97@lists.stanford.edu. To subscribe to the free listserv, send an email to: majordomo@lists.stanford.edu with the following message: Subscribe empowerment-evaluation97@lists.stanford.edu Do not add anything to the message (including thanks) - it is an automated system.
Society for Prevention Research	www.preventionresearch.org/SPR_NPN_Listserv.php
Prevention Connection — The Violence Against Women Prevention Partnership	Prevention Connection's moderated email list (listserv), Prevent-Connect, is a forum to discuss the newest violence against women prevention efforts. Information on how to subscribe to the listserv is available at: http://www.preventconnect.org/display/displaySection.cfm?sectionID=240

Usually, only subscribers to a listserv can post a message to it. You can usually find instructions on how to join a listserv on the website of the organization or association that manages it. If you know someone who already subscribes to a listserv, you can ask him or her to post your announcement or RFP. When an e-mail is sent to the listserv, everyone who subscribes to the listserv will receive it. Some listservs have hundreds or thousands of subscribers.

Because of the volume of e-mail most people receive every day, the subject line of an e-mail often determines whether a recipient opens it. Therefore, consider carefully what you include in the subject line for your job announcement or RFP. Be specific, but concise. For example: "Empowerment evaluator position announcement in Atlanta, GA."

Note from the Field

"Initially, our staff was concerned that we would be unable to find a qualified candidate in our state.... The initial candidates who voiced interest were either unqualified or lived out of state, a major concern considering travel costs within our state. After posting our contract announcement on the American Evaluation Association website, however, we got an immediate inquiry from the woman eventually selected as our evaluator.... Our hiring committee was unanimous in our assessment of our chosen candidate, and honestly felt that we could not have found a better candidate even in a major metropolitan area."

Job banks

In addition to listservs, some associations include job banks on their websites. Consultants and firms will check these sites when seeking work. Table 10 offers a short list of organizations relevant to evaluators and/or violence prevention that include job banks on their websites. Instructions on how to post your job announcement or RFP in the job bank are provided by each website. You may need to register your organization on the website before you can post your announcement or RFP.

Table 10. Job Banks for Locating Potential Empowerment Evaluators

Host Organization of Job Bank	Web Address
American Evaluation Association	www.eval.org/programs/careercenter.asp
American Psychological Association	http://jobs.psyccareers.com
Society for Prevention Research	www.preventionresearch.org/trainingcareershome.php

Other places to post your job announcement

If your organization has its own website, be sure to post your job announcement prominently on the home page. In addition to the Internet, consider state and local newsletters and periodicals that may be relevant to potential empowerment evaluators. For example, some states and communities have associations of nonprofit organizations that may publish a monthly or quarterly newsletter. If your own organization circulates a newsletter, be sure to post your announcement there.

Invite Potential Candidates to Apply

Promising candidates for your empowerment evaluation position may not be actively seeking work when you post your job announcement or RFP, or they may not see the announcement. Therefore, it is wise to proactively seek out and contact potential candidates and let them know about your position.

Resumé banks

Some organizations' websites maintain resume banks and lists of evaluators. The American Evaluation Association maintains a list of evaluators by geographic region (www.eval.org/find_an_evaluator/evaluator_search.asp). The association also links to numerous regional, state, and metro-area affiliate organizations (found at www.eval.org/aboutus/organization/affiliates.asp). Many of these organizations have their own job banks and resume banks.

Universities

Departments of public health, sociology, social work, education, and psychology, as well as university-based research centers, often have faculty who are trained and have experience in evaluation. Start with a list of colleges and universities near you. Identify the relevant academic departments at each school by searching their website. Call the chair of each of those departments and ask for the names of faculty who have experience in evaluation, especially those who teach evaluation.

Partners and other organizations

Call your partners and contacts at nonprofit organizations, coalitions, government agencies, and universities located in your state or local community to ask for the names of good evaluators with whom they have worked.

Funders

Funders are increasingly requiring their grantees to evaluate the program or strategy for which they are provided funding. They may be able to recommend evaluators.

Making contact

Once you have a list of potential candidates, call or e-mail them. Given the high volume of e-mails most people receive, phone calls are more likely to reach potential candidates who are not already familiar with you or your organization.

When contacting potential candidates:

1. Introduce yourself and your organization.

2. Let them know you are looking for an evaluation consultant who can assist your organization in building its evaluation capacity using an empowerment evaluation approach.

3. Ask if you can send them your job announcement.

4. Let them know how to contact you.

5. If given the opportunity, describe the nature of the available position and the length of the project.

6. If they are interested in the position, you may want to have them submit one or all of the following:

    - Letter of interest that summarizes their experience, their interest in the position, and their contractual rate (how much they charge for their work) and whether the rate is firm or negotiable.

    - Resume or curriculum vitae.

    - Proposal describing their approach to completing the tasks in the job announcement.

    - Sample evaluation summaries of past evaluations they have conducted.

    - Letters of reference from other organizations for which they have conducted or been involved with evaluation.

7. Let them know that if they are not interested or available, you would welcome referrals to other professionals who may be qualified and interested.

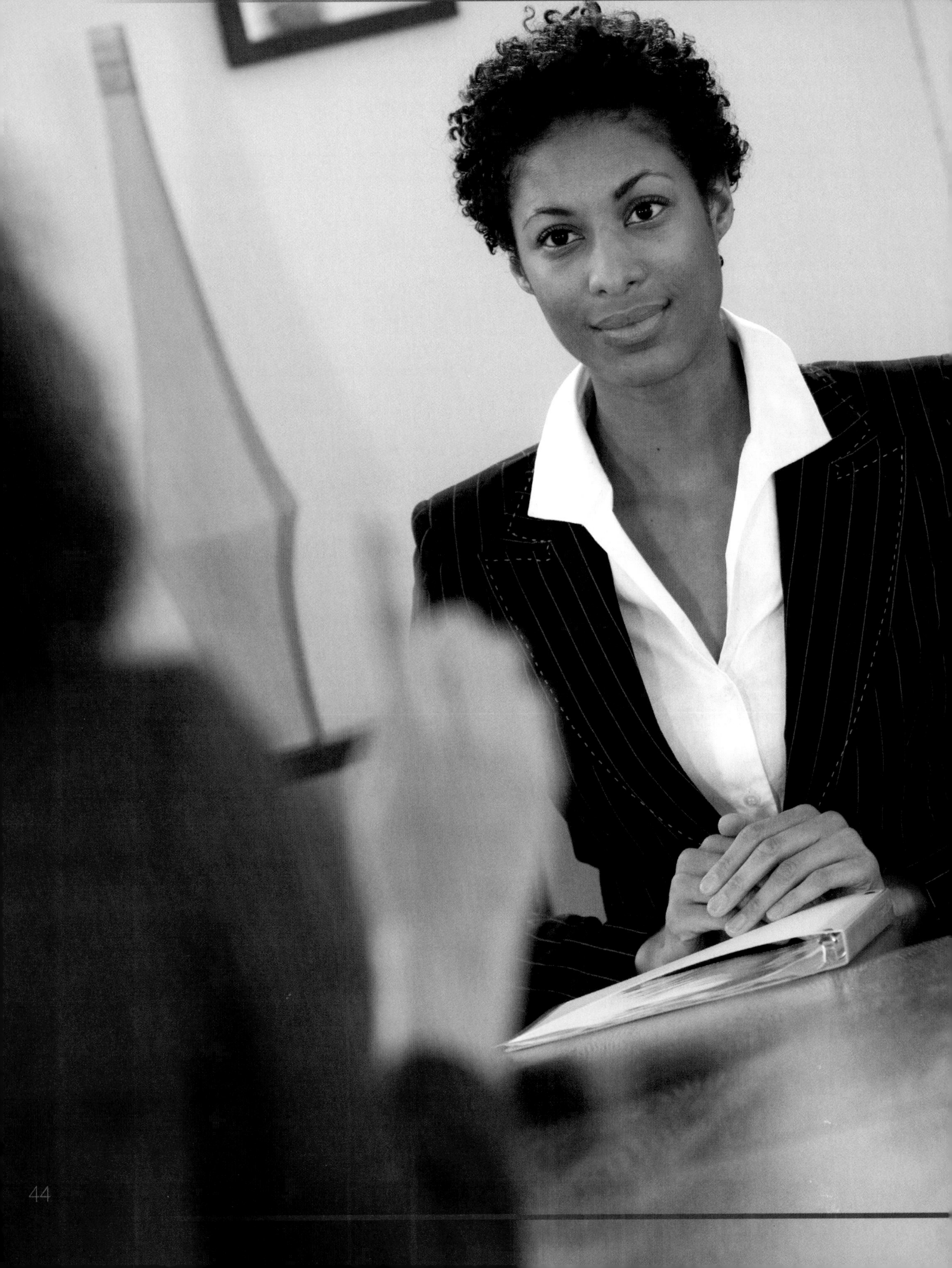

Step 4: Assessing the Candidates

After your deadline for applications has passed, take a look at your pool of applicants. Review letters of interest, resumes, curriculum vitae, and/or proposals you received to assess which of the candidates have met the established qualifications and choose the most desirable candidates to interview.

Review Resumes and Applications

Develop a process for reviewing submitted materials with your hiring committee. Depending on the number of people or organizations that have expressed interest in the position, you may choose to divide the submitted materials among all the members of your hiring committee or have each member of the committee review each applicant's materials. You could choose a block of time to meet as a group and go through all submitted materials together. Follow your organization's required procedure to evaluate each submittal based on the qualifications you specified in your job announcement or RFP. Worksheet 6: Resume Review on page 82 in Appendix B can help with this process. You may need to adapt the worksheet to fit the specific qualifications for your position. When an evaluation team responds to your job announcement or RFP, consider completing a separate resume review worksheet for each member of the team to ensure that your organization's basic requirements for the position are covered by at least one team member or the team as a whole.

Develop an Interview Plan and Conduct Interviews

After the hiring committee has determined which applicants appear to meet your desired qualifications on paper, it's time to interview those candidates. During the interview you will get a sense of what it might be like to work with each candidate and will find out which candidates possess the required knowledge and skills. When conducted well, interviews can reveal candidates' approaches to problems and challenges, their working style, and their communication skills. You can also learn a lot about their comfort and familiarity with empowerment evaluation.

During one of your hiring committee meetings, spend some time planning your interview process. Issues to consider include who will conduct the interviews, how many candidates you will interview, how interviews will be scheduled, and what questions

will be asked (Harding, 2000). Worksheet 7: Interview Plan on page 83 in Appendix B can assist in this process. Each consideration is discussed in further detail below.

Decide who will conduct the interviews

Ideally, every member of your hiring committee will have a role in the interview process. That way, you will have multiple perspectives to consider when making your final decision, rather than relying on one person's opinion of each candidate. Interviews can be conducted by a group, or candidates can be interviewed by one member of the hiring committee at a time.

Note from the Field

"A panel format was used to conduct the interviews. The panel consisted of six individuals including our organization's executive director, the director of the State Department of Health's Division of Injury Prevention Control, the DELTA Program coordinator, the EMPOWER Program coordinator, and two local domestic violence/sexual assault program staff. Thus, our panel reflected the concerns and priorities of funders, program management, program staff, and community stakeholders."

Decide how many candidates to interview

The number of applicants interviewed should be based on the size and quality of your applicant pool. Arbitrarily setting a number in advance could result in interviewing someone who you already know is not qualified or in missing someone who would be a good match for the position.

Notes from the Field

"We interviewed four candidates once. We interviewed three in person and one evaluation team via phone because of their distance from our office."

. . . .

"We selected eight applicants for phone interviews and three for face-to-face interviews."

Decide how interviews will be scheduled

Decide whether you want to schedule interviews back-to-back (on 1 or 2 days) or spread them out over a longer period. Spreading them out may be easier logistically, but it also lengthens the hiring process and increases the possibility of losing a good candidate to another job while the process is being completed.

The hiring committee may choose to have a key member conduct preliminary, informational interviews by phone before inviting candidates for a formal interview. This step allows you to find out more about applicants' qualifications, tell them more about the position, and gauge their interest before you spend your time—and theirs—on a formal interview.

Note from the Field

"Informational interviews were useful for the program coordinator and potential candidates—candidates were better able to gauge if they fit the position, and the coordinator gained practice and confidence in describing the position."

Develop a list of interview questions

To compare candidates, the hiring committee should develop a core set of questions that are asked of every candidate. Questions tailored for each applicant may also be appropriate in order to get a better understanding of their unique skill set and experience as presented on their resume or in their proposal. For both core questions and tailored questions, the hiring committee should be prepared to ask follow-up or probing questions to ensure that the answer provided by a specific candidate actually answers the question or provides the required information. Also, be sure to give the applicant time to ask questions; this is important for the applicant, and it allows you to assess his or her interest in the position.

All interviews should provide an opportunity for each candidate to describe their perspectives on empowerment evaluation. Specifically, candidates can describe their perspectives on the goals, activities, opportunities, and challenges associated with empowerment evaluation. The candidate can also describe how they would go about building individual and organizational evaluation capacity. Interview questions may seek to assess how the candidate understands and supports the three key empowerment evaluation roles: evaluator, organization, and funder. Make sure candidates understand the differences between these roles. A list of sample interview questions is provided on pages 93-94 in Appendix F.

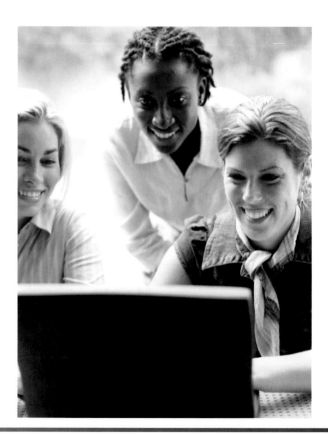

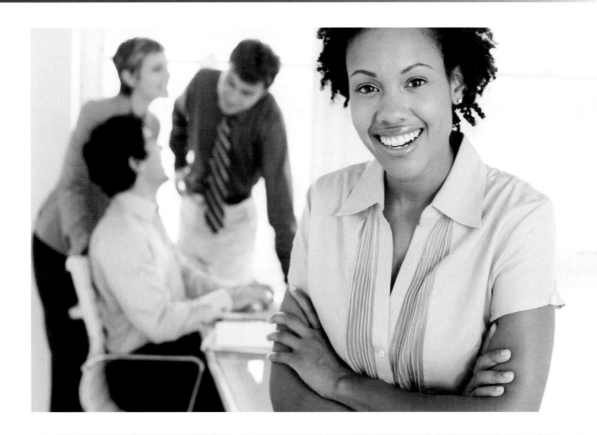

Notes from the Field

"I think our initial evaluator was too steeped in research and traditional evaluation, and we needed more support in evaluation capacity building than she was able to provide. We should have been more upfront in the interview that we wanted an evaluator who could serve as a facilitator to help build community ownership and investment in evaluation and strategy improvement."

. . . .

"Applicants were provided a copy of the interview questions an hour prior to the interview for their preparation. All interviews started with an introduction and overview of our organization,. . .and the program and a description of the interview process and timeline. Each member of the panel then proceeded to take turns asking the applicant questions from the list of interview questions, while the other members of the panel took notes on the applicant's responses. Upon conclusion of the question phase of the interview, each applicant was allowed time to ask questions and/or provide the panel with other information relevant to their experience and qualifications for the position."

Notes from the Field

"We had 16 questions regarding evaluation experience, domestic violence— related work, primary prevention, and experience in training and working with community-based initiatives. Of the 16 questions, two were hypothetical scenarios. All questions were open-ended and we asked follow-up questions for clarity or more information as needed based on the responses that we received."

· ·

"We conducted initial phone interviews and developed a phone interview report for each applicant. The hiring committee reviewed phone interview reports and resumes and selected three candidates for face-to-face interviews.... Applicants were rated using tools from the 'How to Hire an Empowerment Evaluator' tool kit [early draft of this manual], and the top candidate was brought in for an interview with the state DELTA Program team."

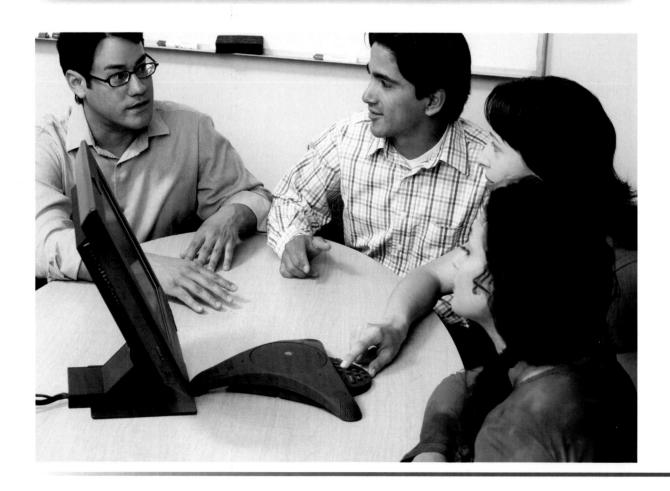

Plan other aspects of the interview

You need not limit your interview process to asking questions. Activities such as taking candidates on a tour of your facilities and/or community and holding a "meet and greet" with other members of your organization or other partnering organizations can help you get to know candidates and help them get to know your organization. You could ask candidates to demonstrate their skills by completing a short writing assignment or interpreting hypothetical evaluation results. Some of the DELTA and EMPOWER Programs asked their candidates to prepare a 10-minute presentation about a particular topic targeted to a local community audience.

Notes from the Field

"The final stage of the interview process was to assess the applicant's writing ability. Applicants were asked to submit a writing sample telling us why they felt they were qualified to the position."

. . . .

"We asked each applicant to write a press release to motivate the community to get involved with local violence prevention efforts and to develop a presentation as if he or she was meeting with a local community-based group. This allowed our organization to assess how the candidate was able to communicate to audiences not familiar with violence prevention and evaluation topics."

Conduct a mock interview before interviewing the first candidate

You might find it useful to have members of your hiring committee practice an interview with a "pretend" candidate before interviewing the actual candidates. This step will help the committee get comfortable with the process and revise interview questions if needed.

Note from the Field

"During the phone interview process, the first candidate was sort of a guinea pig. This person was at a disadvantage because the team learned much about how to improve the process through the experience of her call. A 'mock interview' prior to beginning our phone interviews may have helped us engage each applicant equally."

Interview all members of evaluation teams

If you decide to interview a firm or evaluation team that works as a group, be sure to interview the actual person(s) who would be assigned to your project and not only a sales consultant responsible for obtaining new clients. When interviewing university faculty, ask to interview any graduate students who would be involved in carrying out the project as well. Suggested questions for interviewing evaluation teams are listed on page 94 in Appendix F.

Rate Interview Performance

When conducting interviews, you will receive a great deal of information about each candidate. Using an interview performance rating form can help you capture and organize the information during and/or immediately after each interview. One has been provided for you on page 84 in Appendix B, Worksheet 8: Interview Performance Rating. Your form should allow you to record the quality of applicants' responses and comments during the interview. The form should also allow you to record your observations of each candidate's punctuality, sense of confidence, verbal communication style, and ability to relate easily and comfortably with others. You can adapt the form to match your chosen interview questions and other qualifications of interest.

Review Work Samples

Reviewing work samples can be a useful way to assess a candidate's writing, teaching, and evaluation skills. This activity can be time consuming, so your hiring committee may want to review work samples from only those candidates who are still being considered after the interviews.

Ask the top candidates to provide a work sample that is similar to the kind of products your evaluator will be asked to develop with you and your evaluation team/organization (since in empowerment evaluation, most deliverables will be a joint effort). You may be interested in seeing a training manual or PowerPoint presentation used to train others on evaluation topics or an evaluation report or strategic plan they developed for or with an organization. Assess how well each candidate is able to translate complex evaluation terms into easy-to-understand language. Worksheet 9: Writing Sample Review on page 85 in Appendix B can be used to record your hiring committee's assessment.

Check References

Professional references are an important source of information in the final stages of choosing a candidate for any position. When you have narrowed your search to no more than two or three candidates, ask each candidate to give you at least three professional references, along with contact information. Your organization may also consider asking candidates to sign a release form to allow each reference to speak freely about the candidate's qualifications.

Ideal references may include:
- A faculty member who worked closely with the candidate during his or her academic training (this does not need to be required of well-established professionals).
- A current or former employer or colleague who knows the candidate's skills as an evaluator.
- At least one practitioner (preferably two) from a program or organization with whom the candidate has worked as an evaluator or has worked with to build its evaluation capacity.

It is common practice to call each reference and ask a series of questions about the applicant. You may find it helpful to share the job announcement with the reference, so that he or she can better gauge whether or not the applicant has the necessary

skills and demeanor to fulfill the requirements of the position. When speaking to references, look for issues that did not emerge during other portions of the application process; references may express reservations about an applicant or provide a more balanced description of an applicant's strengths and weaknesses. References can also help your hiring committee confirm or solidify its own impressions of the applicant, allowing your team to have greater confidence in its decision.

Some questions you may want to ask references are:
- How long have you known the applicant? What was the nature of your work together?
- What is it like to work with the applicant?
- How does he or she set priorities? How does he or she work with others?
- How would you describe the applicant's strengths and challenges as an evaluator?
- The applicant is applying for an empowerment evaluator position. He or she will work as a coach to build evaluation capacity within our organization; he or she will give up control over many of the decisions in the evaluation process. Have you observed the applicant in this type of role before? If so, how did he or she manage that role? If not, how do you think he or she would manage that kind of role?
- How would you describe the candidate's skills and effectiveness in training and technical assistance?
- How would you describe the candidate's ability to facilitate group discussions to reach decisions where the members of the group may have very divergent priorities?
- How would you describe the candidate's ability to follow through on deliverables?
- Do you have any concerns about recommending the applicant for this position?

Select the Best Candidate(s)

As you near the end of your interview process, one candidate may emerge as the best choice, and your organization may be ready to extend an offer with little deliberation. However, decisions do not always come this easily. You may have more than one excellent candidate to choose from, or you may have to weigh the strengths and limitations of each candidate. In making these tough decisions, it is helpful to consolidate the information you have from each part of the application and interview process into a single summary form for each candidate. Worksheet 10: Candidate Summary on page 86 and Worksheet 11: Candidate Ranking onpage 87 in Appendix B may be helpful in selecting the top candidate(s).

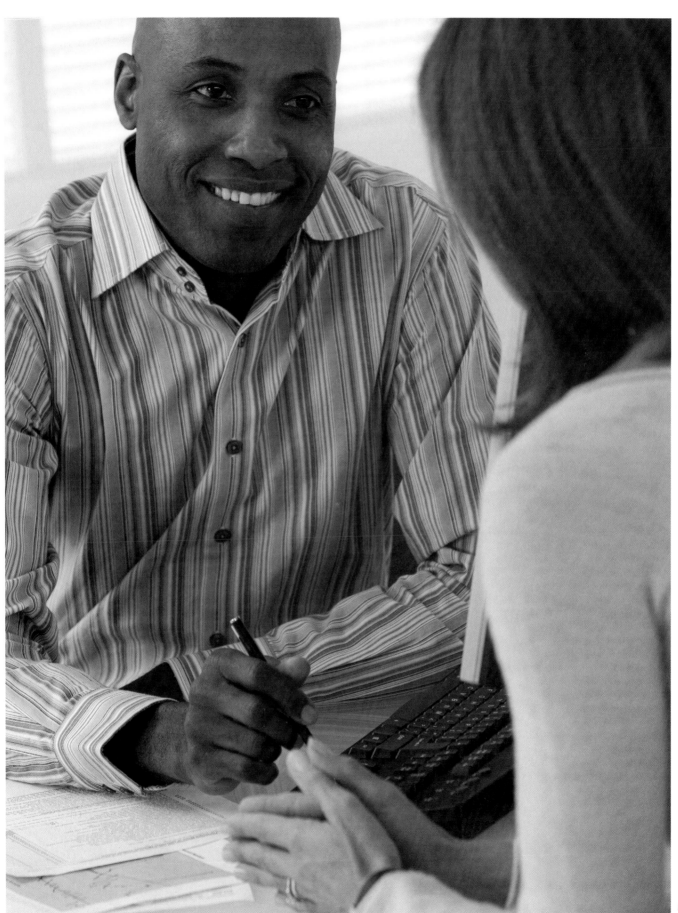

Notes from the Field

"We engaged the committee in a consensus-building process by first narrowing the field from four to three candidates. Then we began listing on a white board the qualifications we were most looking for and rated the candidates. After that, we began polling committee members about their first and second choices so we could gauge where the group was. Consensus emerged within 45 minutes. We agreed on a first and second choice. Each committee member was given the right to block the decision if they felt it necessary. No one blocked or stood aside during the decision-making process."

"We had two candidates who had extensive background in evaluation, domestic violence—related work, primary prevention, and experience in training and working with community-based initiatives. The deciding factors were the level of education and prior experience specifically with CDC projects."

"One candidate received higher ratings by some hiring committee members because she had adequate evaluation experience, but also had several years experience working with a local rape crisis center. The other candidate was rated higher by other committee members because she had a great deal more experience single-handedly managing evaluation projects, had used…empowerment evaluation previously, and had many years experience working with community groups made up of very diverse individuals (different socioeconomic, educational, racial and ethnic backgrounds) with successful outcomes… However, she did not have experience working on the issue of sexual violence…. One key question…was, "Which candidate brings more to the state prevention team that is currently missing from the team?" Since many members of the state prevention team have a great deal of experience working with sexual violence issues, the candidate with the strongest evaluation and community experience was the obvious choice."

Make a Job Offer

Once your hiring committee selects your top candidate, your organization is ready to make a job offer. Decide who within the organization is the most appropriate person to extend an offer— the executive director, human resources director, or the program manager. Common practice is to notify the candidate of the offer by phone and follow up with a formal letter that documents the job offer. Depending on the candidate's response and your budget, you may need to negotiate the rate until it is acceptable to both the candidate and your organization.

Be prepared for the possibility that your top candidate may decline the position. In this case, you will want to extend an offer to your second-choice candidate, and possibly to a third-choice candidate. Wait to notify any qualified candidates that your position has been filled until after a candidate has accepted your offer.

Note from the Field

"Three applicants emerged as possible candidates, all with various levels of expertise. A decision was made fairly easily by consensus of the group based on the candidate's expertise in domestic violence and research. However, after further discussion with the candidate, she decided that it was not a good fit for her because she had never done an actual "evaluation," although her past work mirrored the chosen planning process in many ways. A second and equally good choice was offered the position, and she too decided the contract would not be something she could take on due to previous obligations and other grant work at her university. Our third candidate accepted our offer and the hiring committee felt satisfied that she is an excellent choice, based on her extensive evaluation experience and openness to using the planning process and the empowerment evaluation principles. The candidate we finally hired actually has the most experience with this approach

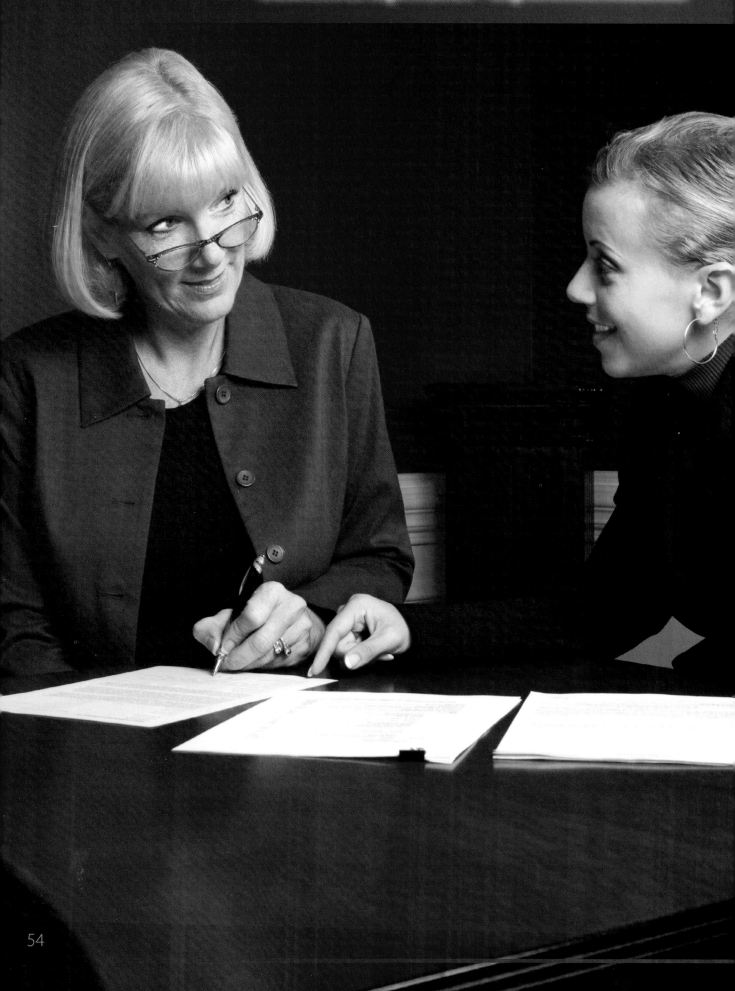

Step 5: Writing An Evaluation Contract

An evaluation contract is a legal agreement between your organization and your chosen candidate about the work to be completed and the compensation to be provided in return. It describes clearly what you expect from your evaluator and what your evaluator can expect from you. And it provides protection for your organization and the evaluator if problems arise. Table 11 lists a number of basic contractual elements (Harding, 2000).

Table 11. Common Elements of an Evaluation Contract

- Agency name and address
- Evaluator name, address, affiliation, and Social Security number
- Person from agency responsible for monitoring the contract
- Scope of work
- Key deliverables (e.g., reports and products) and due dates
- Duties and responsibilities
- Required progress reports and meetings, including attendance at trainings or conferences
- Payment amount, payment schedule, and conditions of payment
- Liability release
- Materials provided to the evaluator by the organization
- Any special terms or conditions, including those for terminating the contract (especially for performance issues)
- A "key personnel" clause if working with a consulting firm or evaluation team
- Statement about confidentiality of the data (e.g., Human Subjects/Internal Review Board processes and approval)
- Data ownership and publication rights
- Restrictions on publishing or presenting evaluation findings
- Signature and date for both organization representatives and evaluator

If your organization is hiring an empowerment evaluator as a staff member, then you'll follow its standard procedures for extending an offer and determining a salary. This section provides an overview of key contracting issues that need to be considered in any contracting process and can inform an organization's existing contracting procedures, whether the organization is a government agency or private not-for-profit.

Unexpected delays and challenges can arise while writing a contract. Be sure to build in plenty of time for this process; then, if you run into roadblocks, your timeline will not be thrown off course.

Notes from the Field

"The contracting process took longer than we had initially expected and required much more "back and forth" negotiation than we had anticipated. . . . As we are technically contracted with a university, it created additional contractual complexities—the selected evaluator and coalition staff would find they were in agreement on a contractual draft, only to have it refused by the university non-evaluator staff. The contracting process was definitely the longest and most labor-intensive part of the contract award process."

"Designing the contract forced us to be very strategic about timeframe, traveling, and budget issues. The negotiations, however, went very smoothly."

"The contracting process was somewhat unwieldy. First, because of the bureaucracy of being a university-affiliated, community-focused organization, the evaluation team uses memoranda of understanding (MOU) instead of contracts and refers to awards as 'grants.' This was not evident until almost the end of the contract process as the budget side of the organization is handled by individuals other than the evaluators. This created issues in terms of format, compliance with CDC guidelines, and potential legal enforcement if problems arose at a later date. We eventually created an MOU that greatly resembles a contract. Final struggles revolved around content for the contract/ MOU as this was the first time our organization had utilized an outside evaluator. Much time was spent by the program coordinator and the coalition attorney drafting a document that was not unnecessarily complicated but provided protection for potential disputes.

Define the Scope of Work and Deliverables

The scope of work and list of deliverables should be designed to serve a well-defined purpose or need, usually building the evaluation capacity of an organization and coaching the organization through an evaluation of a specific strategy. As you specify each task, responsibility, or deliverable in the contract, continuously ask yourselves how that task or deliverable relates back to your main purpose or goal for hiring an empowerment evaluator. You can use the list of responsibilities and deliverables specified in your job announcement or RFP as a starting point.

Members of your organization will share responsibility with your empowerment evaluator for building the evaluation capacity of your organization and in planning and conducting an evaluation of a specific strategy. Therefore, the evaluation contract should describe how your evaluator will "assist," "coach," "support," and "inform" your capacity-building efforts and your initial evaluation. You want to avoid statements like "The evaluator will plan and

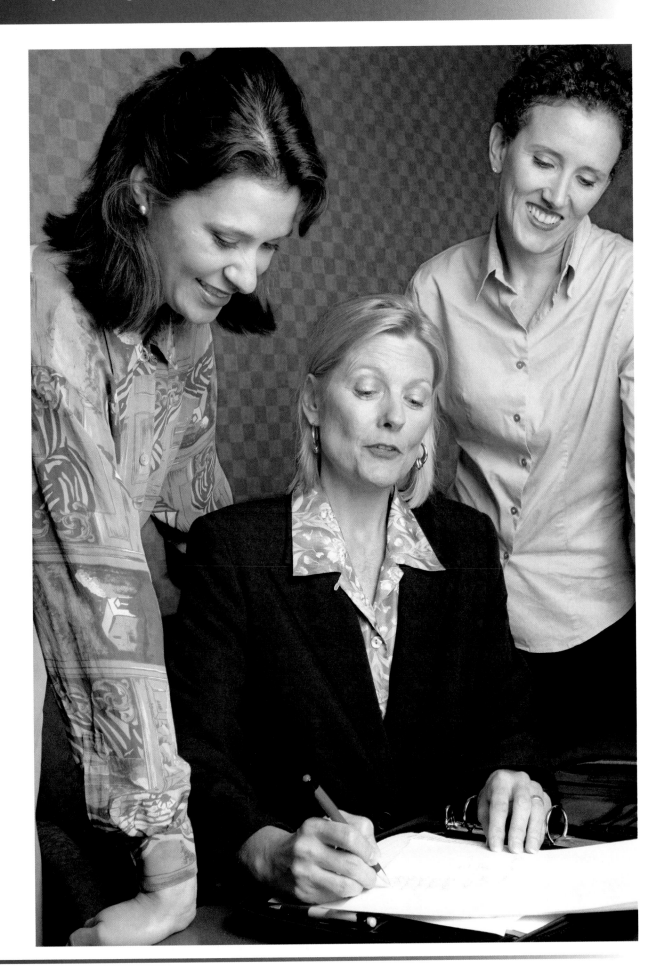

conduct an evaluation of the strategy" because such language does not reflect the principles of empowerment evaluation. It is appropriate to require your evaluator to submit progress reports about his or her role in promoting and fulfilling the purpose and scope of work of your contract. However, if you want to uphold the principles of empowerment evaluation, the evaluator should not be solely responsible for building your organization's evaluation capacity or for any evaluation conducted. The due dates for each task and/or deliverable should be explicit in the contract.

Define a Payment Rate and Schedule

There are different ways to arrange payment in an evaluation contract. A "fixed price contract" is when you pay a certain fee for a certain scope of work over a period of time. In this arrangement, the evaluator agrees to fulfill the stated responsibilities, tasks, and deliverables in the contract over a specified time period (typically 1, 3, or 6 months) for a fixed amount, regardless of the amount of time required to complete the individual tasks. When using a fixed price contract, you and your evaluator should estimate the amount of time expected to fulfill the scope of work and then calculate the fixed amount based on an agreed upon rate of pay. The benefit of this approach is that you can be certain from the outset how much the evaluation will cost for a given period. The downside is, if you greatly overestimate or underestimate the amount of time necessary to do the work, you could end up paying more or less than is appropriate.

Another type of contract is a "time and materials contract." In this arrangement, you agree to pay an established rate for the evaluator's time and other resources used. Evaluators charge different rates for their time depending on their education and level of experience. Hourly rates may range from $50 to $100 an hour; daily rates may range from $300 to $800 or higher. Some evaluators may lower their rate for time-intensive projects. The evaluator will typically send a monthly or quarterly invoice to your organization detailing the hours spent in that period and a total amount due. This arrangement can be useful when you expect the amount of time the evaluator spends on the project to vary from month to month. It allows payment to match the ebb and flow of the work. On the other hand, if the evaluator ends up spending much more time on the project than you anticipated, the cost of the evaluation could be higher than you had planned. To protect your budget, you can specify a monthly, quarterly, or yearly limit. For example, when specifying the rate of pay in the contract, you would add "…not to exceed $_____ over a 6-month period."

Your organization may also consider including a phased-work plan in the contract. Under such a plan, the empowerment evaluator must complete satisfactory work and submit acceptable deliverables for a given phase before beginning work included in the next phase.

Be aware of extra fees when contracting with a university or research firm

If you choose to work with an evaluator from a university or an evaluation firm, you may be charged indirect fees by the university or firm in addition to the rate charged by the evaluator or evaluation team. In some cases, you may have the option of contracting directly with the individual evaluator rather than with the university or corporate entity to avoid these fees. In other cases, professionals may be legally bound to work only through their affiliate organization.

Indirect fees are used to pay utilities, office space, office supplies as well as support the university's or firm's infrastructure, such as libraries and information technology systems. These fees can range from 15% to more than 50% of the base cost of a given contract. Do not assume that the initial fee quote is non-negotiable. Sometimes fees designed for large, federal research grants are quoted for nonprofit contracts by mistake; more appropriate fee structures may be available for smaller, nonprofit organizations.

If you work for a government agency, you may want to investigate if your agency has a standing agreement with the particular university regarding its indirect fee rate.

Develop a Budget for Other Expenses

After developing a payment rate and schedule and negotiating indirect fees, you and your empowerment evaluator will need to develop a budget that covers expenses other than the evaluator's hourly rate and indirect fees. Such costs can include travel expenses, communication costs, and office supplies. A sample budget is provided on page 95 in Appendix G; although it is for an evaluation team, the budget categories also apply to working with a single evaluator.

Specify Personnel When Contracting with an Evaluation Team

If you are contracting with an evaluation team from a university or research firm, be sure to include clear language in your contract about who will be working on your evaluation contract and in what roles. Frequent and unnecessary changes in the members of your evaluation team can disrupt the momentum of capacity building and prevent the kind of relationship building that facilitates good empowerment evaluation. Therefore, you want to specify under what conditions evaluation team members may change or be replaced so that such changes do not occur without your prior knowledge and consent. Consider including a "key personnel" clause to your contract such as the one that follows.

Sample "Key Personnel" Clause

The individuals identified below are considered essential to the work being performed under this contract. Substitution, or substantial reduction in their efforts, shall not be made without prior written approval of [Organization]. In the event of the continued unavailability of designated personnel or personnel acceptable to [Organization], [Organization] shall have the right to terminate this contract.

Designated Key Personnel:
[name(s) of key person(s)]

Specify Data and Product Ownership

Your organization and your empowerment evaluator will need to specify who owns the data and products developed during the empowerment evaluation process. In some cases, your organization may wish to specify that the data and results produced through the empowerment evaluation process will belong to your organization. In this case, your contract should include a clause that requires your evaluator to obtain prior approval before using data from the evaluation in conference presentations or professional publications. In other cases, you and your empowerment evaluator may want to share ownership of data and products developed, with each party having certain rights and responsibilities.

State Conditions for Termination and Steps to Address Performance Issues

The evaluation contract should include a clause that allows your organization to terminate the contract if the evaluator is not fulfilling your evaluation needs. A progressive course of action may be outlined in the contract regarding poor performance; this action plan should be reviewed in the initial orientation with the empowerment evaluator. Also, your organization may decide to have a general termination clause in the contract and work with the empowerment evaluator early in the process to develop a progressive course of action regarding performance.

Have an Attorney Review Your Contract

Have an attorney review your contract to ensure that your organization is fully protected. If you work for a government organization, your legal department will probably be required to review any contract before it is signed by all parties.

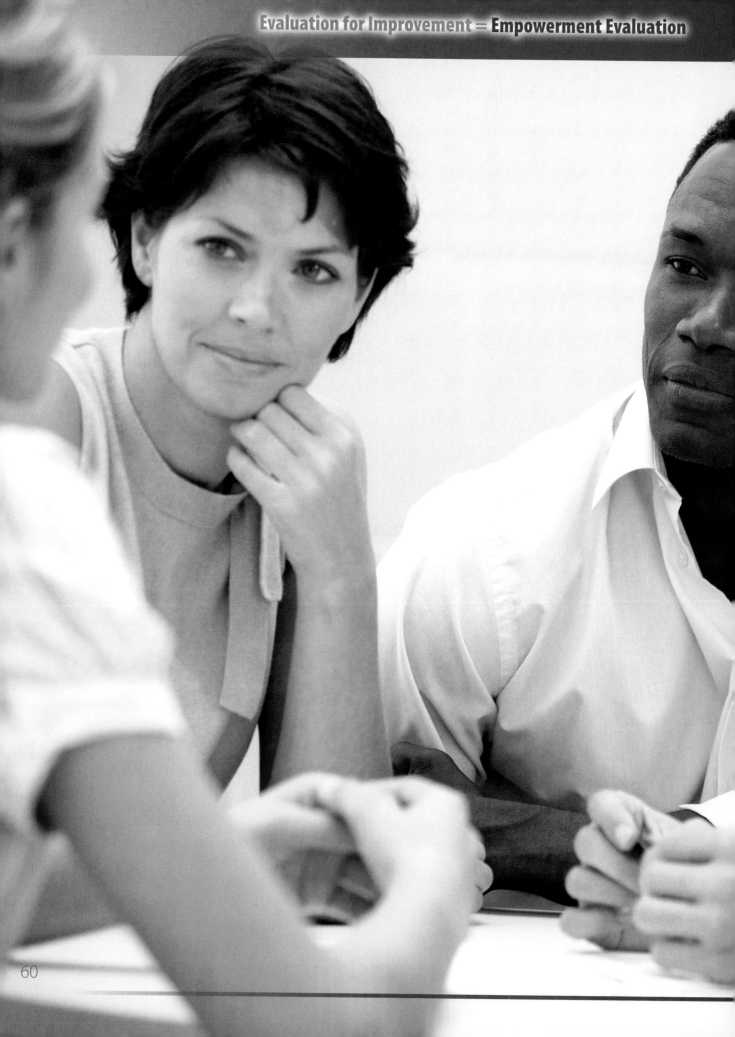

Step 6: Building an Effective Relationship With Your Evaluator

To build an effective working relationship with your evaluator, you will need to establish an empowerment evaluation team; exchange information, including expectations of and experiences with evaluation; define roles and responsibilities; and establish a process and schedule for communication. You'll also need to outline a process to address any problems that arise with your evaluator's performance. This section describes each of these steps in detail.

Establish an Empowerment Evaluation Team

Your empowerment evaluator is an evaluation coach (if you hired an evaluation team, you have a group of evaluation coaches), and a coach works with a team. Your empowerment evaluation team should be made up of key members of your organization who will be involved in the inner workings of building evaluation capacity and conducting an initial evaluation of a strategy. It should also include key individuals who are directly involved in developing and implementing the initial strategy to be evaluated. An ideal size for an evaluation team is four to six individuals.

Not everyone in your organization can be on the evaluation team. However, all members of your organization, and your key stakeholders, should be aware of the intent to build organizational evaluation capacity through the "learn-by-doing" process of evaluating the organization's strategies to assess if they are achieving their stated goals and outcomes. Often the "learn-by-doing" process is initiated by the organization selecting one particular strategy to evaluate to see if it is achieving its stated goals and outcomes. Other strategies may be evaluated at a later date as organizational evaluation capacity increases. Organizational members and stakeholders should have input into any evaluations and be informed of the evaluation results and their implications. You can include input from other members of your organization and other stakeholders through focus groups, quarterly meetings, and trainings.

Conduct an Orientation for the Evaluation Team

An orientation session is an excellent way for members of the evaluation team to exchange information relevant to building the evaluation capacity of the organization and evaluating a specific strategy. It allows the entire evaluation team to get on the same page regarding the purpose of the empowerment evaluation process, evaluation team, and the contract with the empowerment evaluator. The orientation session may take place in one day or over several days or weeks.

During orientation, your organization may provide the evaluator with information such as:

- History of your organization, including its history with evaluation
- Organization's mission statement
- Organization's current strategic plan
- Organizational chart
- Job descriptions
- Copies of grant proposals and requirements from funders
- Notes or materials from your organization's discussion regarding its readiness to participate in an empowerment evaluation process (see Step 1, pages 23–26)
- Copy of this manual
- Documents (e.g., grants, progress reports, any previous evaluations) related to the initial strategy to be evaluated

Your organization may also ask the evaluator to attend key organizational and partnership meetings, tour your facilities, and meet with staff and possibly service recipients.

As part of this orientation process, the evaluator may provide the organization with a more in-depth description of empowerment evaluation—including key lessons, successes, and challenges from the literature and an overview of his or her experience with evaluation in general and empowerment evaluation specifically.

Given that a main component of empowerment evaluation is capacity building, this orientation session should include discussions with key organizational staff regarding current evaluation capacity of both individuals and the organization. The orientation process will allow the empowerment evaluator to assess both facilitators and barriers to building organizational evaluation capacity and make recommendations for how to build organizational evaluation capacity.

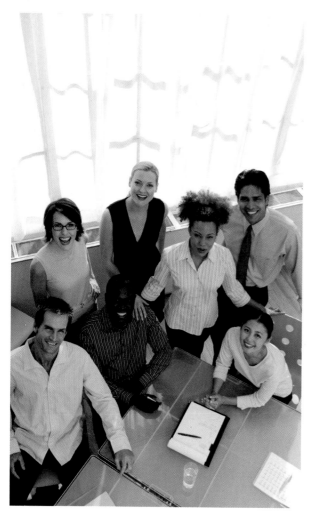

Establish Roles

As noted earlier, there are three major roles defined within empowerment evaluation: the evaluator, the organization, and the funder. It is important to establish up front how each empowerment evaluation team member fits into these roles and into the collaborative process that is empowerment evaluation. Who does what, when, how, and to what standards?

Over time, roles may change. For instance, the empowerment evaluator may initially facilitate training and technical assistance. Later, as the organization's evaluation capacity increases, organizational staff may co-facilitate these activities with the

empowerment evaluator. If roles change as capacity increases, they need to be openly redefined so that all team members know who is doing what. Thus, role clarification and re-clarification may be ongoing.

Defining roles may initially pose a significant challenge, but it is also an opportunity for team members to build cohesion and a vision for their work. It is also a time to address similar and different work styles and find ways to minimize conflict among the work styles. Defining roles in a group setting can ensure that each person understands, rather than assumes, what the roles and responsibilities of the other team members are and where roles may overlap. Extra effort is needed to determine processes for handling overlapping roles and responsibilities.

Part of establishing roles includes creating a clear process for making decisions that reflects the empowerment evaluation principles. Thus, your empowerment evaluation team should have a substantial discussion about what types of decisions will be made by whom and under what circumstances. Once agreed upon, these decision-making protocols should be written up and distributed to all empowerment evaluation team members. The decision-making protocols may need to be modified as the evaluation capacity building process proceeds to take into consideration new information or changes in roles and responsibilities among team members.

Establish a Communication Schedule

Set up a communication and meeting schedule. Do you need to have weekly, biweekly, or monthly meetings of the evaluation team? Will minutes be kept, and if so, by whom? Do you need to set up weekly phone contact between the evaluator and the project director in addition to regular meetings? Is there an efficient way to communicate with all members of the evaluation team by e-mail? Be willing to make changes to the communication plan as needed.

Review Contract Information Regarding Performance Issues

Performance issues may include a breakdown in communication, lack of follow through, failure to provide deliverables on time, poor quality of work, and actions in clear contradiction to the empowerment evaluation principles. The organization's expectations in each of these areas need to be clearly expressed to

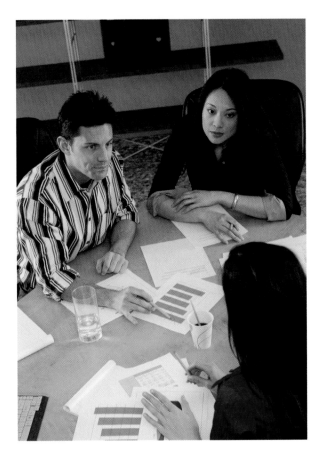

Have a plan for when things go wrong

When performance issues do arise, your organization should address them as quickly as possible. An honest, open dialogue within the evaluation team may be appropriate in some cases; in other cases, a meeting between the organization's main contact and the evaluator may be more appropriate in order to communicate the seriousness of the performance issue.

Performance issues may stem not from the evaluator, but from the organization's growing pains in integrating evaluation into its daily activities. Campbell et al. (2004) noted that even after initial orientation meetings, some staff were still confused about the role of the empowerment evaluator. Some staff still thought the empowerment evaluator was hired as an external evaluator to assess the organization's strategies rather than build the organization's evaluation capacity to evaluate its own strategies through a learn-by-doing process. In this instance, the organization's unwritten expectations of the evaluator did not match the written expectations in the evaluation contract. Continued open dialogue about expectations and empowerment evaluation may help with this issue.

In some cases, the evaluator may realize that he or she likes leading and conducting independent evaluations more than teaching or building evaluation capacity according to empowerment evaluation principles. These evaluators are good to keep in mind should your organization ever want to complement its empowerment evaluation work with independent evaluation.

Overall, it is important to review the contract and deliverables in an honest, open dialogue to ensure that everyone is in agreement about the deliverables, the processes used to reach those deliverables, and the parties responsible for producing them. Such a dialogue may reveal that the organization and evaluator have different understandings of these issues that cannot be reconciled. In that case, part ways amicably. On the other hand, such a dialogue may re-energize both parties.

the evaluator, and the evaluator needs to acknowledge that he or she understands these expectations.

A progressive course of action to address performance issues may be developed collaboratively by your organization and the empowerment evaluator. It's good to have a regular mechanism for check-in and assessment by all involved, perhaps as part of the communication schedule. This regular check-in should assess progress on deliverables and meeting the work plan.

Note from the Field
"As with any consultant, there will be a period of learning. To address this learning curve and prevent larger problems later, attend to misunderstandings immediately in a constructive, collaborative manner."

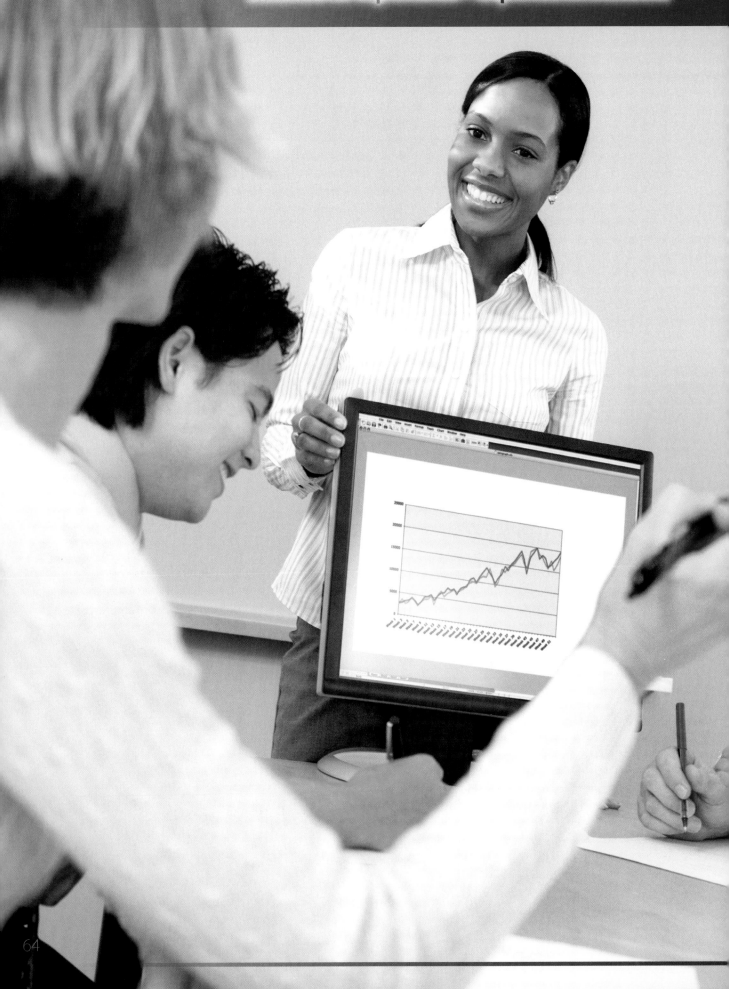

Step 7: Assessing and Sustaining the Evaluation

Once your empowerment evaluation process is underway, periodically assess whether the process is meeting your organization's needs and accomplishing its purpose—which is ultimately to help your organization build its evaluation capacity so that it can assess whether or not its strategies are achieving their stated goals and outcomes. Your first such assessment should occur early in the process so you can identify and address problems before they become more difficult to resolve.

Make Sure You Are Really Doing Empowerment Evaluation

Even when all parties agree to do empowerment evaluation, it can still be easy to slip into more independent evaluation roles in which the evaluator conducts the evaluation and reports findings back to the organization and stakeholders who implement the strategy. Stakeholders may find that they have so much to do just in implementing a strategy and doing their "regular" work that it is easier to let the evaluator do the evaluation work. Evaluators can also stray from the principles when they assume too much control over the evaluation process and do not facilitate enough ownership among organizational staff. When this happens, many of the benefits of empowerment evaluation are lost. If the empowerment evaluation activities are not building the organization's ability to integrate evaluation within the organization, then it is not really empowerment evaluation.

The best way to ensure that your organization reaps the benefits of empowerment evaluation is to be confident that your entire evaluation team is working in a way that is consistent with the 10 principles of empowerment evaluation. Keep the principles visible by posting them in your meeting space, handing them out at your meetings, and putting them on the cover of your evaluation notebook. Pick one principle to discuss at each of your evaluation meetings and ask what you could be doing to better promote that principle in your work together.

To help you stay on track, assess how each major stakeholder in your evaluation is maintaining the empowerment evaluation principles. You can do this early in your evaluation process as a baseline measurement, and continue to make periodic assessments to measure your progress over time (e.g., every 6 or 12 months).

To do a quantitative assessment, you can use a rating scale like the one suggested in Worksheet 12: Empowerment Evaluation Principles Role Assessment located on page 88 in Appendix B. You can use the role descriptions provided on pages 18–21 (Tables 2–4) as a guide to complete the scale. You can also adapt Worksheet 12 or create your own. To collect more in-depth information, you can conduct interviews and/or focus groups with your key stakeholders about the evaluation process to learn more about how they are maintaining the empowerment evaluation principles.

As you assess your use of the empowerment evaluation principles, do not expect perfection. Miller and Campbell (2006) reviewed 47 empowerment evaluation case examples published in the literature and found very few case examples that adhered to all 10 principles. Rather, most of the case examples indicated that they were consistent with 4 to 7 of the empowerment evaluation principles. Six empowerment evaluation principles—community ownership, inclusion, democratic participation, community knowledge, evidence-based strategies, and accountability—may be practiced and observed earlier in the empowerment evaluation process than the four principles of improvement, social justice, capacity building, and organizational learning. Your organization may want to use the four latter principles as indicators as to whether or not the empowerment evaluation process is having an impact on your organization. Is your organization more focused on improvement after working with an empowerment evaluator for 6 months than it was before? After 6 months of working with an empowerment evaluator, what types of individual and organizational capacity have been built? Has your organization's culture increased its focus on learning from mistakes? Is your organization now more dedicated to social justice activities than it was before working with an empowerment evaluator?

Continue the Evaluation Process After the Evaluation Contract Ends

Empowerment evaluation is a long-term investment. That investment only pays off if you sustain empowerment evaluation as an ongoing process after your initial contract with your empowerment evaluator ends. A major goal of empowerment evaluation is to make evaluation a part of your daily operations. The key to sustaining empowerment evaluation is in building organizational evaluation capacity. The greater that capacity at the end of an evaluation contract, the less dependent you will be on outside consultants to meet your future evaluation needs. Start thinking now about how you can sustain your evaluation process after your empowerment evaluation contract ends.

Note from the Literature

Foundation for the Future, which coordinates a range of services to families in Spartanburg, South Carolina, provides an excellent example of how to sustain empowerment evaluation over time (Keener, Snell-Johns, Livet & Wandersman, 2005). After 2 years of doing empowerment evaluation, a key staff member of the organization had developed sufficient capacity to conduct a number of evaluation tasks independent of the evaluator. To reflect the change in her role and responsibilities, the organization changed her job title from Collaboration Manager to Director of Collaboration and Evaluation. Eventually, the individual holding this position needed to leave her position. Before hiring someone to replace her, the organization considered the skills that were needed to carry on the evaluation tasks that the current employee had acquired over time. The new evaluation tasks were included in the job description, and the organization selected a new employee with an appropriate educational background and skill set to carry out the tasks. The departing employee provided hands-on training to the new employee. The first evaluation report prepared by the new Director of Collaboration and Evaluation was equal in quality to those of the previous Director of Collaboration and Evaluation. The staff transition was a seamless process that ensured no organizational evaluation capacity was lost.

The note from the literature illustrates the development of both individual and organizational evaluation capacity. Regarding individual capacity, one particular employee was able to take on new evaluation tasks over time so that she could eventually do them with little help from the evaluator and in collaboration with other stakeholders. To build individual evaluation capacity, staff members are typically given tools, training, and technical assistance to acquire new knowledge, skills, and motivation to use evaluation tools and methods. Individuals also need to have the resources necessary to do evaluation work (e.g., time, computer equipment and software, survey instruments).

Fortunately, the organization described in the note from the literature did not stop its organizational capacity building efforts after it developed significant evaluation capacity among one particular employee, the Director of Collaboration and Evaluation. Its leaders recognized that people come and go from organizations, and that if they did not integrate their employee's new skills within the organization, the employee's evaluation capacity would simply go away when she left the organization. By changing the title of a key position to reflect evaluation and collaboration, which is essential within empowerment evaluation, and by incorporating evaluation skills and tasks into the position's job description, the

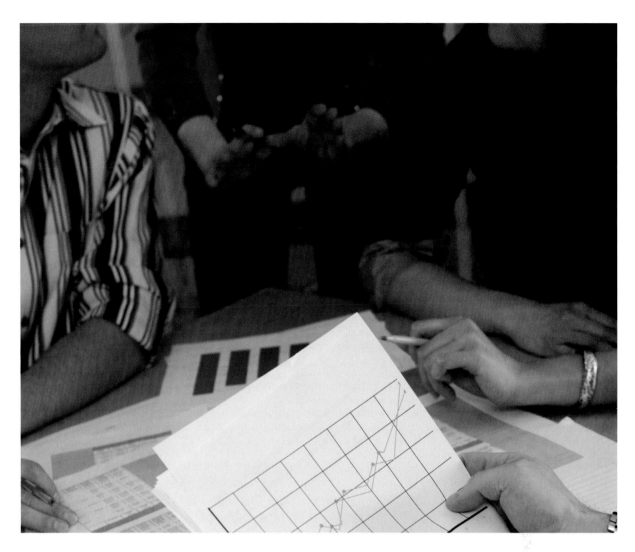

organization took a significant step in sustaining organizational evaluation capacity. An additional significant step would be to incorporate the practice of empowerment evaluation principles into every staff members' job description.

Specifically, evaluation capacity can be integrated into your organization's structures, processes, resources, and priorities. Consider including evaluation activities in the job descriptions of various staff members. Assess staff members' performance related to the evaluation activities included in their job descriptions during annual reviews and establish regular, perhaps monthly, meetings to review evaluation results and make recommendations for improvement. Offer regular training and technical assistance to address the various evaluation activities for which the employees are responsible. Seek funding streams that support evaluation within the organization, and dedicate staff, management, and board time to developing evaluation skills and establishing evaluation processes. Finally, prioritize the integration of evaluation into regular programmatic activities within your organization rather than viewing evaluation as a luxury or add-on feature.

Campbell and colleagues (2004) conducted a study to find out whether sexual assault programs that participated in an empowerment evaluation project were still doing evaluation after the project ended. Follow-up phone interviews were conducted with 10 prevention programs and 24 victim service programs. The study found that 90% of the programs were still doing evaluation about one year after the formal empowerment evaluation project had ended and that all of the programs had made changes in their policies and procedures based on the results of their evaluation findings. Perhaps what is most remarkable about these findings is that, because of staff turnover, only 8 of the 34 program staff interviewed had worked with the empowerment evaluation project. Even so, the new staff members were familiar with the project and referred specifically to tools that they still use from the project. These findings suggest that these sexual assault programs were successful in building and sustaining organizational evaluation capacity through an empowerment evaluation process.

Glossary

Child maltreatment

Any act or series of acts of commission or omission [that results in harm, potential for harm, or threat of harm to a child. Physical abuse, sexual abuse, psychological abuse, and neglect are specific forms of child maltreatment (Leeb, Paulozzi, Melanson, Simon & Arias, 2008).

Cultural competence

A developmental process that results in individual, community, and organizational understanding of cultural differences and similarities within, among, and between communities, cultures, and populations. This competence requires drawing on the community-based values, traditions, and customs to work with knowledgeable persons of, and from, specific populations in developing specific strategies and communications to address their needs (Cross et al.,1989; National Center for Cultural Competence, n.d.; Pyles & Kim, 2006).

Effectiveness

The positive outcomes of a strategy, program, or policy derived under real-world conditions, such as limited resources for materials and training and limited control over factors affecting implementation (Flay et al., 2005)

Efficacy

The positive outcomes of a strategy, program, or policy derived under optimal or ideal conditions of delivery, such as having adequate resources, well-trained and supervised personnel, and control over factors affecting implementation (Flay et al., 2005)

Empowerment evaluation

An evaluation approach that provides program stakeholders with tools for program planning, implementation, and self-evaluation and integration of evaluation into the planning and management of the program or organization for the purpose of increasing the likelihood that programs will achieve their intended outcomes (Wandersman et al., 2005).

Evaluation

The systematic collection of information about the activities, characteristics, and outcomes of strategies (i.e., programs) to make judgments about the strategy, improve strategy effectiveness, and/or inform decisions about future strategy development (U.S. DHHS, 2005).

Individual evaluation capacity

The extent to which individuals have the knowledge, skills, resources, and motivation to plan, conduct, analyze, and use evaluation.

Intimate partner violence (IPV)

Physical, sexual, or psychological harm by a current or former intimate partner. IPV can occur among heterosexual or same-sex couples and does not require sexual intimacy. The four categories of IPV are physical violence, sexual violence, threat of physical or sexual violence, and psychological/emotional abuse (including coercive tactics) (Saltzman, Fanslow, McMahon & Shelley, 1999).

Organization

A coalition, partnership, local or state government agency, or nonprofit agency and its respective stakeholders.

Organizational evaluation capacity

The extent to which a given organization has the structures, resources, processes, and motivation to plan, conduct, analyze, and use evaluation (Gibbs, Napp, Jolly, Westover & Uhl, 2002; Torres & Preskill, 2001).

Outcome evaluation

The systematic collection of information to assess the impact of a strategy or program, present conclusions about its merit or worth, and make recommendations about future strategy or program direction or improvement (U.S. DHHS, 2005).

Participatory evaluation

Evaluation that involves collaborative work with the individuals, groups, or communities who have a decided stake in the program development (Cousins & Whitmore, 1998).

Primary prevention Approaches that aim to prevent violence before it occurs (Dahlberg & Krug, 2002).

Process evaluation The systematic collection of information to document and assess how a particular program or strategy was implemented and operated (U.S. DHHS, 2005)

Program The combination of several strategies designed to deliver reinforcing messages to one intended population in a variety of settings (Powell , Dahlberg, Friday, Mercy, Thornton, & Crawford, 1996).

Protective factor An attribute, situation, condition, or environmental context that buffers or moderates the effect of risk (US DHHS, 2001).

Research Using scientific methods, standards (e.g., internal and external validity), and designs (e.g., experimental design that uses a control group) to evaluate the **efficacy** or effectiveness of a strategy, program, or policy (U.S. DHHS, 2005)

Risk factor An attribute, situation, condition, or environmental context that increases the chances of a person behaving violently or experiencing violence (U.S. DHHS, 2001).

Sexual violence Completed or attempted sex acts against the victim's will or involving a victim who is unable to consent, abusive sexual contact, and non-contact sexual abuse, including sexual harassment and stalking (Basile & Saltzman, 2002).

Social ecological model A multi-level model that suggests human behavior (e.g., violence) is the result of the complex interplay of individual, relationship, community, and societal factors (Dahlberg & Krug, 2002).

Stakeholders The persons or organizations having an investment in what will be learned from an evaluation and what will be done with the knowledge (U.S. DHHS, 1999).

Strategy A set of activities that, together, are intended to reduce violent behavior, such as social skills training, mentoring, social marketing, or policy changes (Powell et al., 1996). These multiple activities together are intended to achieve goals or results at a specific level of the social ecology.

Suicide and Suicidal Behavior Suicidal behavior exists on a continuum from thinking about ending one's life (i.e., suicidal ideation), to developing a plan, to nonfatal suicidal behavior (i.e., suicide attempt), to ending one's life (suicide) (CDC, n.d.).

Youth violence The intentional use of physical force or power, threatened or actual, exerted by or against children, adolescents, or young adults (ages 10–29) that results in or has a high likelihood of resulting in injury, death, psychological harm, maldevelopment, or deprivation (Mercy, Butchart, Farrington, & Cerda, 2002).

References

Basile, K. C., & Saltzman, L. E. (2002). *Sexual violence surveillance: uniform definitions and recommended data elements version 1.0.* Atlanta: Centers for Disease Control and Prevention, National Center for Injury Prevention and Control.

Brennan Ramirez, L. K., Baker, E. A., Metzler, M. (2008). Promoting Health Equity: A resource to help communities address social determinants of health. Atlanta: Department of Health and Human Services, Centers for Disease Control and Prevention.

Campbell, R., Dorey, H., Naegeli, M., Grubstein, L. K., Bennett, K. K., Bonter, F., et al. (2004). An empowerment evaluation model for sexual assault programs: Empirical evidence of effectiveness. *American Journal of Community Psychology, 34,* 251–262.

Centers for Disease Control and Prevention [CDC]. (1999). Framework for program evaluation in public health. *Morbidity and Mortality Weekly Report, 48*(RR-11). Atlanta, GA: Centers for Disease Control and Prevention.

Centers for Disease Control and Prevention [CDC]. (no date). *Suicide Prevention, Scientific Information: Definitions.* Retrieved April 30, 2008 from http://www.cdc.gov/ncipc/dvp/Suicide/Suicide-def.htm.

Chinman, M., Imm, P., & Wandersman, A. (2004). *Getting to outcomes 2004: Promoting accountability through methods and tools for planning, implementation, and evaluation.* Santa Monica, CA: RAND Corporation.

Cook, T. D., & Shadish, W. R. (1987). Program evaluation: the worldly science. *Evaluation Studies Review Annual, 12,* 31–70.

Cross, T., Bazron, B., Dennis, K., & Isaacs, M. (1989). *Towards a culturally competent system of care: A monograph on effective services for minority children who are severely emotionally disturbed: Volume I.* Washington, DC: Georgetown University Child Development Center.

Cousins, J. B., & Whitmore, E. (1998). Framing participatory evaluation. *New Directions for Evaluation, 80,* 5–23.

Dahlberg, L. L., & Krug, E.G. (2002). Violence—a global overview. In E. G. Krug, L. L. Dahlberg, J. A. Mercy, A. B. Zwi & R. Lozano (Eds.), *World Report on Violence and Health* (pp. 1-21). Geneva, Switzerland: World Health Organization.

Dugan, M. A. (1996). Participatory and empowerment evaluation. In D. M. Fetterman, S. J. Kaftarian & A. Wandersman (Eds.), *Empowerment evaluation: Knowledge and tools for self-assessment and accountability* (pp. 277–303). Thousand Oaks, CA: Sage Publications.

Fetterman, D. M. (1982). Ibsen's baths: Reactivity and insensitivity (A misapplication of the treatment-control design in a national evaluation). *Educational Evaluation and Policy Analysis, 4*(3), 261–279.

Fetterman, D. M. (1994). Empowerment evaluation [American Evaluation Association presidential address]. *Evaluation Practice, 15* (1), 1–15.

Fetterman, D. M. (2001a). Empowerment evaluation and self-determination: A practical approach toward program improvement and capacity building. In N. Schneiderman, M. A. Spears, J. M. Silva, H. Tomes & J. H. Gentry (Eds.), *Integrating behavioral and social sciences with public health* (pp. 321–350). Washington, DC: American Psychological Association.

Fetterman, D. M. (2001b). *Foundations of empowerment evaluation.* Thousand Oaks, CA: Sage Publications.

Fetterman, D. M. (2005). Empowerment evaluation principles in practice: Assessing levels of commitment. In D. M. Fetterman & A. Wandersman (Eds.), *Empowerment evaluation principles in practice* (pp. 42–72). New York: Guilford Press.

Flay, B., Biglan, A., Boruch, R., Castro, F., Gottfredson, D., Kellam, S., et al. (2005). Standards of evidence: Criteria for efficacy, effectiveness and dissemination. *Prevention Science, 6,* 151–175.

References

Gibbs, D., Napp, D., Jolly, D., Westover, B., & Uhl, G. (2002). Increasing evaluation capacity within community-based HIV prevention programs. *Evaluation and Program Planning,* 25, 261–269.

Harding, W. (2000). *Locating, hiring, and managing an evaluator.* Newton, MA: CSAP's Northeast Center for the Application of Prevention Technologies.

Joint Committee on Standards for Educational Evaluation. (1994). *The program evaluation standards* (2nd ed.). Thousand Oaks, CA: Sage Publications.

Keener, D. C., Snell-Johns, J., Livet, M., & Wandersman, A. (2005). Lessons that influenced the current conceptualization of empowerment evaluation: Reflections from two evaluation projects (pp. 73–91). In D. M. Fetterman & A. Wanderman (Eds.), *Empowerment evaluation principles in practice.* Thousand Oaks, CA: Sage Publications.

Leeb, R. T., Paulozzi, L., Melanson, C., Simon, T., & Arias, I. (2008). *Child maltreatment surveillance: Uniform definitions for public health and recommended data elements, version 1.0.* Atlanta, GA: Centers for Disease Control and Prevention, National Center for Injury Prevention and Control.

Livet, M., & Wandersman, A. (2005). Organizational functioning: Facilitating effective interventions and increasing the odds of programming success. In D. M. Fetterman & A. Wandersman (Eds.), *Empowerment Evaluation Principles in Practice* (pp. 123–154). New York: Guilford Press.

Mayer, S. E. (1996). Building community capacity with evaluation activities that empower. In D. M. Fetterman, S. J. Kaftarian & A. Wandersman (Eds.), *Empowerment evaluation: Knowledge and tools for self-assessment and accountability* (pp. 332–378). Thousand Oaks, CA: Sage Publications.

Mercy, J. A., Butchart, A., Farrington, D., and Cerda, M. (2002). Youth Violence. In E. G. Krug, L. L. Dahlberg, J. A. Mercy, A. B. Zwi, & R. Lozano (Eds.), *World Report on Violence and Health* (pp. 25-56). Geneva: World Health Organization.

Miller, R. L., & Campbell, R. (2006). Taking stock of empowerment evaluation: An empirical review. *American Journal of Evaluation,* 27(3), 296–319.

National Center for Cultural Competence. (n.d.). *Conceptual frameworks/models, guiding values and principles.* Retrieved April 5, 2008, from Georgetown University Center for Child and Human Development Web site http://www11.georgetown.edu/research/gucchd/nccc/foundations/frameworks.html.

Powell, K. E., Dahlberg, L. L., Friday, J., Mercy, J. A., Thornton, T., & Crawford, S. (1996). Prevention of youth violence: rationale and characteristics of 15 evaluation projects. *American Journal of Preventive Medicine,* 12(Suppl.), 3–12.

Preskill, H. & Torres, R. T. (1999). *Evaluative inquiry for learning in organizations.* Thousand Oaks, CA: Sage Publications.

Pyles, L., & Kim, K. M. (2006). A multilevel approach to cultural competence: A study of the community response to underserved domestic violence victims. *Families In Society,* 87, 221–229.

Rossi, P. H., & Freeman, H. E. (1989). *Evaluation: A systematic approach* (3rd ed.). Newbury Park, CA: Sage.

Rossi, P. H., Freeman, H. E., Lipsey, M. W. (1999). *Evaluation: A systematic approach* (6th edition). Thousand Oaks, CA: Sage.

Saltzman, L. E., Fanslow, J. L., McMahon, P. M., & Shelley, G. A. (1999). *Intimate partner violence surveillance: Uniform definitions and recommended data elements,* version 1.0. Atlanta (GA): Centers for Disease Control and Prevention, National Center for Injury Prevention and Control.

Schnoes, C. J., Murphy-Berman, V., & Chambers, J. M. (2000). Empowerment evaluation applied: Experiences, analysis, and recommendations from a case study. *American Journal of Evaluation,* 21(1), 53–64.

Torres, R. T., & Preskill, H. (2001). Evaluation and organizational learning: Past, present, future. *American Journal of Evaluation,* 22(3), 387–395.

U.S. Department of Health and Human Services [U.S. DHHS] (2001). *Youth Violence: A Report of the Surgeon General.* Washington, DC:U.S. Government Printing Office.

U. S. Department of Health and Human Services [U.S. DHHS]. (2005). *Introduction to program evaluation for public health programs: A self-study guide.* Atlanta, GA: Centers for Disease Control and Prevention.

University of Texas – Houston Health Science Center, School of Public Health (1998). *Practical evaluation of public health programs.* Atlanta, GA: Centers for Disease Control and Prevention. Retrieved April 30, 2008, from http://www.cdc.gov/eval/workbook.PDF

Wandersman, A. & Snell-Johns, J. (2005). Empowerment evaluation: clarity, dialogue, and growth. *American Journal of Evaluation,* 26(3), 421-428.

Wandersman, A., Snell-Johns, J., Lentz, B. E., Fetterman, D. M., Keener, D. C., Livet, M., et al. (2005). The principles of empowerment evaluation. In D. M. Fetterman, & A. Wandersman (Eds.), *Empowerment evaluation principles in practice* (pp. 27–41). New York: Guilford Press.

Weaver, L. & Cousins, J. B. (2004). Unpacking the participatory process. *Journal of Multidisciplinary Evaluation,* 1, 19–40.

Appendix A: Resources for General Evaluation and Empowerment Evaluation

General Evaluation

American Evaluation Association

www.eval.org

This website includes listings and links for a variety of evaluation resources and networks.

Centers for Disease Control and Prevention (CDC) Resources

1. CDC Evaluation Working Group Homepage

www.cdc.gov/eval/index.htm

This website provides an overview of the work of the CDC Evaluation Working Group and its effort to promote evaluation in public health. Specific information on this website includes an overview of the working group, highlights of CDC's framework for program evaluation, and additional resources that may help when applying the framework.

2. *Framework for Program Evaluation in Public Health*

www.cdc.gov/eval/framework.htm

This website outlines CDC's evaluation framework.

3. *Introduction to Program Evaluation for Public Health Programs: A Self-Study Guide*

www.cdc.gov/eval/evalguide.pdf

This document is a "how to" guide for planning and implementing evaluation activities. The manual is based on CDC's Framework for Program Evaluation in Public Health and is intended to assist state, local, and community managers and staff of public health programs in planning, designing, implementing, and using the results of comprehensive evaluations in a practical way. The strategy presented in this manual will help ensure that evaluations meet the diverse needs of internal and external stakeholders, including assessing and documenting implementation, outcomes, efficiency, and cost-effectiveness, and taking action based on evaluation results to increase impact.

4. Practical Evaluation for Public Health Programs

www.cdc.gov/eval/evalguide.pdf

Designed for non-statisticians, this course will enable participants to learn 1) why evaluation and building commitment for it are important; and 2) how to design and conduct practical and effective evaluation in a team environment. Learners will be introduced to and work through the CDC evaluation framework.

Community Tool Box

http://ctb.ku.edu

This website offers resources related to program planning and evaluation, suitable for community groups and others.

David Fetterman

www.stanford.edu/~davidf/empowermentevaluation.html

This webste includes information and links relevant to empowerment evaluation.

Evaluation Exchange

www.gse.harvard.edu/hfrp/eval/issue27/index.html

This website features an online evaluation journal.

Getting To Outcomes 2004

www.rand.org/publications/TR/TR101/

This website contains a manual providing a 10-step framework for planning, implementing, and evaluating prevention programs. Although the manual is geared to substance abuse prevention, but the framework can be applied to any type of prevention.

Empowerment Evaluation

Campbell, R., Dorey, H., Naegeli, M., Grubstein, L. K., Bennett, K. K., & Bonter, F., et al. (2004). An empowerment evaluation model for sexual assault programs: Empirical evidence of effectiveness. *American Journal of Community Psychology,* 34, 251–262.

Cousins, J. B., & Whitmore, E. (1998). Framing participatory evaluation. *New Directions for Evaluation,* 80, 5–23.

Fetterman, D. M. (2001). *Foundations of empowerment evaluation.* Thousand Oaks, CA: Sage Publications.

Fetterman, D. M., Kaftarian, S., & Wandersman, A. (Eds.). (1996). *Empowerment evaluation: Knowledge and tools for self-assessment and accountability.* Thousand Oaks, CA: Sage Publications.

Fetterman, D. M., & Wandersman, A. (2005). *Empowerment evaluation principles in practice.* New York: Guilford Press.

Fetterman, D. M, & Wandersman, A. (2007). Empowerment evaluation: Yesterday, today, and tomorrow. *American Journal of Evaluation,* 28, 179–198.

Linney, J. A., & Wandersman, A. (1996). Empowering community groups with evaluation skills: The Prevention Plus III Model. In D. Fetterman, S. Kaftarian, & A. Wandersman (Eds.), *Empowerment evaluation: Knowledge and tools for self-assessment and accountability* (pp. 259–276). Thousand Oaks, CA: Sage Publications.

Livet, M., & Wandersman, A. (2005). Organizational functioning: Facilitating effective interventions and increasing the odds of programming success. In D. M. Fetterman & A. Wandersman (Eds.), *Empowerment evaluation principles in practice* (pp. 123–154). New York: Guilford Press.

Miller, R. L. (2005). *Empowerment evaluation principles in practice,* edited by David M.Fetterman and Abraham Wandersman, reviewed by Robin L. Miller. *Evaluation and Program Planning,* 28, 317–319.

Miller, R. L., & Campbell, R. (2006). Taking stock of empowerment evaluation: An empirical review. *American Journal of Evaluation,* 27(9), 296–319.

Schnoes, C. J., Murphy-Berman, V., & Chambers, J. M. (2000). Empowerment evaluation applied: Experiences, analysis, and recommendations from a case study. *American Journal of Evaluation,* 21(1), 53–64.

Scriven, M. (1997). Empowerment evaluation examined. *Evaluation Practice,* 18(2), 165–175.

Stockdill, S. H., Baizerman, M., & Compton, D. W. (2002). Toward a definition of the ECB process: A conversation with the ECB literature. *New Directions for Evaluation,* 93, 7–25.

Wandersman, A., & Snell-Johns, J. (2005). Empowerment evaluation: Clarity, dialogue, and growth. *American Journal of Evaluation,* 26(3), 421–428.

Zimmerman, K., & Erbstein, N. (1999). Promising practices: Youth empowerment evaluation. *Evaluation Exchange,* 5(1).

Appendix B: Worksheets for Hiring an Empowerment Evaluator

This appendix contains 12 worksheets to help your organization work through the process of hiring an empowerment evaluator. Each worksheet can be tailored to fit the needs of your organization and/or hiring process. For more information about each of these worksheets, look back at the step and page referenced below regarding where the worksheet was discussed in a particular step and where it can be found in the Appendix.

Worksheets Specifically Tailored to the Seven-Step Process	Discussed on Page	Found in Appendix on Page
Step 1—Worksheet 1. Resources for Empowerment Evaluation	26	76
Step 1—Worksheet 2. Hiring Committee Checklist	27	78
Step 1—Worksheet 3. Tracking Progress for Hiring an Empowerment Evaluator	29	79
Step 2—Worksheet 4. Defining Job Responsibilities and Deliverables	32	80
Step 2—Worksheet 5. Defining Qualifications of the Position	34	81
Step 4—Worksheet 6. Resume Review	45	82
Step 4—Worksheet 7. Interview Plan	45	83
Step 4—Worksheet 8. Interview Performance Rating	49	84
Step 4—Worksheet 9. Writing Sample Review	50	85
Step 4—Worksheet 10. Candidate Summary	50	86
Step 4—Worksheet 11. Candidate Ranking	50	87
Step 7—Worksheet 12. Empowerment Evaluation Principles Role Assessment	65	88

Worksheet 1. Resources for Empowerment Evaluation

Resources for empowerment evaluation are not limited to funding. Also take into account the knowledge, attitudes, skills, experience, and time available within your existing staff. Consider those who have previous experience with evaluation, data entry skills, survey administration skills, etc. Take stock of supplies and equipment that may be needed for evaluation activities, such as computers, software, printers, copiers, etc.

Funding for evaluation usually comes from grants that support the development, implementation, and/or evaluation of a particular strategy. Many federal grants now suggest or require that a percentage of the funds be used for evaluation; some grants also specify a minimum and maximum percentage of funds to be spent on evaluation. List the financial resources you have available for building the evaluation capacity of your organization and for evaluating specific strategies. As noted in Table 4 on page 21, Role of the Funder in an Empowerment Evaluation, ideally funders would provide not only money, but also moral support, tangible guidance, and active engagement in building evaluation capacity within an organization and in evaluating any specific strategies.

An example of a completed worksheet appears on the next page.

Staff knowledge, attitudes, skills, experience, and time

Financial resources
Can be used to build organizational evaluation capacity in general:

Must be used only to evaluate a specific strategy:

Supplies and materials

Contextual Resources (e.g., local university, existing partnerships)

Example:
Worksheet 1. Resources for Empowerment Evaluation

Staff knowledge, attitudes, skills, experience, and time

1. Program coordinator has data entry skills. She has used these skills to develop reports to all funders, following each funder's unique format. She understands how to conduct a quality check to ensure that the data were accurately entered in the database.

2. Program coordinator and manager have analytical skills. Each month, these two staff members review reports going to funders to assess the progress of the strategies funded. Through their efforts, several key actions have been taken over the past year to improve strategy implementation, recruiting efforts, and community mobilization efforts.

3. Various staff members have voiced enthusiasm about being able to know if their strategies are working and being able to report that to funders and the community.

4. Funding from the EZ Pillar Foundation will allow both the program coordinator and program manager to devote 15% (6 hours) of their time each week to empowerment evaluation activities.

Financial resources

Can be used to build organizational evaluation capacity in general:

1. Alota Mulla Foundation: 5% of annual grant ($5,000)

2. EZ Pillar Foundation: 10% of annual grant ($25,000)

3. United Way: 5% of annual award ($10,000)

Must be used only to evaluate a specific strategy:

4. State Department of Health: 5% of annual award ($20,000)

Supplies and materials

1. Donated computer and printer from XYZ Corporation

2. Donated software from Office Warehouse

3. Office space for empowerment evaluator – 2 days a week

Contextual Resources (e.g., local university, existing partnerships)

1. Statistics professor at local university has offered to provide, at no cost, a student intern for 10 hours per week to assist in data collection, entry, and analysis and to personally assist in developing process and outcome measures for the strategy to be evaluated.

2. Local organization that has used an empowerment evaluator previously has offered to share training and technical assistance materials used by their empowerment evaluator to reduce the resources needed to develop materials for this organization.

3. Local evaluation association has offered to do a presentation on the various types of evaluation and what organizational evaluation capacity is and how it is developed.

4. State sexual assault coalition has used an empowerment evaluation approach and is available to provide feedback, encouragement, and support to the organization. The coalition has offered to have quarterly conference calls to help address any issues that may arise. As not many organizations have worked to build their own evaluation capacity, the state sexual assault coalition hopes to offer a normative perspective of the rewards and challenges of this approach.

Worksheet 2. Hiring Committee Checklist

Our hiring committee includes:

❏   The executive director or program manager of our organization (or someone in another leadership position).

(Name)_____

❏   The staff member who will directly supervise the work of the evaluator.

(Name)_____

❏   A staff member who has responsibility for and leadership over the programs/strategies being addressed
by the empowerment evaluation (if applicable).

(Name)_____

❏   A front-line staff member who implements the program/strategy that will be evaluated (if applicable).

(Name)_____

❏   A representative of partner organizations or local organizations that will be working with our
empowerment evaluator (if applicable).

(Name)_____

❏   An individual with evaluation knowledge and experience (internal or external to organization).

(Name)_____

❏   Other (Please list):

❏   All members of our hiring committee have signed a confidentiality agreement to protect the privacy of our applicants.
An example of a confidentiality agreement is in Appendix C, on page 89.

Worksheet 3. Tracking Progress for Hiring an Empowerment Evaluator

Key tasks for hiring	Plan to complete this task			
	What needs to be done?	**Who will do it?**	**Target date**	**Date done**
Form hiring committee				
Write job announcement (see Appendix D on page 90 for example)				
Post job announcement				
Identify and contact potential candidates				
Review resumes and select candidates for interviews				
Conduct interviews of top candidates				
Request and review work samples from top candidates				
Conduct a meet and greet of top candidates				
Check references of select candidates				
Select candidate and make a job offer				
Develop and sign an evaluation contract with chosen empowerment evaluator				

Worksheet 4. Defining Job Responsibilities and Deliverables

Our empowerment evaluator will have responsibilities related to the following grants or funding sources...

Responsibilities in building evaluation capacity will include...

Our empowerment evaluator will assist in completing the following reporting requirements...

Facilitation responsibilities will include . . .

Travel requirements will include...

Our empowerment evaluator will help us establish the following ongoing evaluation processes...

Other...

Worksheet 5. Defining Qualifications of the Position

Qualification Area	Minimum qualifications	Preferred qualifications
Education/ training		
Previous work experience		
Orientation to evaluation		
Facilitation skills		
Communication and interpersonal skills		
Other qualifications		
Other considerations		

Worksheet 6. Resume Review[10]

	Rating			
Qualifications[11]	**0** **Not Sure**	**1** **Does not meet minimum requirements**	**2** **Meets minimum requirements**	**3** **Exceeds minimum requirements**
Educational/training background (Minimum requirement: Masters Degree)				
Course work in statistics and research methods (Minimum requirement: 12 hours of statistics and research methods)				
Previous professional evaluation experience (Minimum requirement: 2 years of participatory/community-based evaluation)				
Orientation to evaluation (Minimum requirement: Views evaluation as a tool for strategy improvement and is enthusiastic about using an empowerment evaluation approach)				
Facilitation Skills (Minimum requirement: is developing the ability to facilitate a group decision-making process in accordance with the 10 empowerment evaluation principles)				
Communication skills (Minimum requirement: Strong verbal and written communication skills)				
Experience working with violence prevention organizations. (Minimum requirement: 2 years)				
Experience working with organizations focused on prevention. (Minimum requirement: 2 years)				
Experience working with diverse community coalitions and/or collaborative partnerships (Minimum requirement: 2 years)				
Experience conducting training with adult learners (Minimum requirement: 2 years)				

Note additional comments on back of worksheet...

Based on review of resume, this candidate: ❑ Exceeds / ❑ Meets / ❑ Does not meet minimum qualification requirements

Total Score _____ **Request an interview?** ❑ Yes ❑ No

---

[10] Adapted from a form developed by the Wisconsin Coalition Against Domestic Violence.

[11] See Table 8. Suggested Qualifications for an Empowerment Evaluator on page 35.

Worksheet 7. Interview Plan

Who will conduct the interviews?

How many candidates will you interview?

How and when will interviews be scheduled?

What questions will be asked?

Will there be additional aspects to the interview other than questions and answers?

Will a mock interview be conducted before the actual candidates are interviewed?

Worksheet 8. Interview Performance Rating[12]

Candidate: _____ Date: _____ Interviewer: _____

Interview Question / Task	Rating 1–4: 1 = marginal, 4 = excellent	Comments
1. (Example) What about this position is most attractive to you? What do you believe will be most challenging about the position for you? (insight / fit / interest in the position)		
2.		
3.		
4.		
5.		

Observational Ratings		
Punctuality		
Sense of confidence		
Verbal communication skills		
Relates comfortably with others		
Demonstrates understanding and value of empowerment evaluation principles throughout responses		
Other:		

[12] Adapted from the North Dakota Council on Abused Women's Services/Coalitions Against Sexual Assault.

Worksheet 9. Writing Sample Review[13]

Candidate _____ Reviewer: _____

What was candidate's role in writing report?

- ☐ Lead
- ☐ Assist
- ☐ Part of Team

Rating

Quality of Writing Sample	0 Not Sure	1 Poor/ Nones	2 Fairs	3 Goods	4 Great	5 Super
Writing skills Report is engaging, clear, and easy to read; writing style is professional; grammar and spelling are correct.						
Organization Report is organized in sections with clear and logical headings; table of contents and appendices are included; report is visually pleasing and easy to follow.						
Substance/Content The report provides meaningful information and recommendations; terms and concepts are well defined (low use of jargon); a take-home message is evident in the report.						
Methodology Report describes an appropriate evaluation design, data collection methods, data analysis, and interpretation of results; report is methodologically accurate.						

Comments:

[13] Adapted from Wisconsin Coalition Against Domestic Violence.

Worksheet 10. Candidate Summary

Candidate: _____

Phone: _____ E-mail: _____

Education Level: _____ Field of Study: _____

Source of Information

Qualification	Resume (Total score)	Interview (Total score)	Work Sample (Total score)	References (Total score)	Total
General evaluation (knowledge, skills, ability)					
Empowerment evaluation (knowledge, skills, ability, inclination)					
Violence prevention Specify area: _____ (knowledge and commitment)					
Communication skills (Verbal and written)					
Work ethic					
Interpersonal skills					
Other					

Total Score:

Worksheet 11. Candidate Ranking

Candidate Finalists	Total Score	Rank
1.		
2.		
3.		
4.		
5.		
6.		
7.		
8.		

Worksheet 12. Empowerment Evaluation Principles Role Assessment[14]

Rate the extent to which each participant of your evaluation process is working consistently with each of the empowerment evaluation principles

1 = **Work is not at all consistent with the principle**
3 = **Work is somewhat consistent with the principle**
5 = **Work is fully consistent with the principle**

Participant	Role Description Am I...	Rating Low High
Evaluator	1. serving as a coach rather than a controller of the evaluation? (community ownership)	1 2 3 4 5
	2. helping the organization internalize the goals, processes, and desired outcomes of its programs and strategies? (improvement)	1 2 3 4 5
	3. supporting the use of organizational and community knowledge in building evaluation capacity and evaluating specific strategies? (community knowledge)	1 2 3 4 5
	4. providing training and technical assistance to the organization to help build the organization's evaluation capacity? (capacity building)	1 2 3 4 5
	5. helping the organization interpret and use data to inform decision making and to make evaluation part of the planning and management of the organization? (organizational learning)	1 2 3 4 5
	Average Rating:	
Organization	1. working closely with the evaluator and using the evaluation process to improve our organization's evaluation capacity and performance? (improvement)	1 2 3 4 5
	2. assuming responsibility for the oversight and direction of the evaluation capacity-building process and evaluations of specific strategies? (community ownership)	1 2 3 4 5
	3. facilitating an environment in which the voices of all stakeholders are equally valued, shared, and heard? (democratic participation)	1 2 3 4 5
	4. using my knowledge of community context, demographics, and conditions to choose prevention goals and strategies and to interpret evaluation findings? (community knowledge)	1 2 3 4 5
	5. creating an organizational climate that is conducive to institutionalizing and learning from evaluation? (organizational learning)	1 2 3 4 5
	Average Rating:	
Funder	1. providing the financial support needed for intensive individual and organizational evaluation capacity building and evaluation? (improvement)	1 2 3 4 5
	2. respecting the autonomy of the organization? (community ownership)	1 2 3 4 5
	3. working with the organization to measure and report the results of the capacity-building efforts and to use evaluation results to improve strategies? (accountability)	1 2 3 4 5
	4. recognizing and validating the use of organizational and community knowledge in planning and evaluation? (community knowledge)	1 2 3 4 5
	5. encouraging the adaptation of evidence-based strategies to the local community context and conditions when appropriate? (evidence-based strategies)	1 2 3 4 5
	Average Rating:	

[14] See Tables 2-4 on pages 18-21 that describe the roles of the organization, evaluator and funder in Empowerment Evaluation.

Appendix C: Sample Hiring Committee Confidentiality Statement[15]

Empowerment Evaluator Search

As an individual involved in the search for an empowerment evaluator for [organization], I recognize and accept my responsibility to protect the confidentiality of every prospect and candidate, the search process itself, and the deliberations of the search committee.

To the degree that I will have access to confidential information and materials related to the search, and with full knowledge of the critical importance of confidentiality to the integrity and success of the search process, I hereby agree:

1. The deliberations of the hiring committee and any and all information relating to such deliberations, and all documents relating to the search and the work of the hiring committee are confidential.

2. Hiring committee chair [name] may disclose the process and status of the hiring committee's work to the public as appropriate.

3. I will not, unless otherwise directed or approved by the committee, disclose confidential information to any person or entity, other than a hiring committee member or a person otherwise designated by the committee chair, or as may be required pursuant to any court order. However, I may disclose information about the process and status of the hiring committee's work which has been disclosed by the committee chair.

4. Requests for information related to the selection and appointment of an empowerment evaluator for [organization] should be directed to the chair of the hiring committee.

5. The obligation to maintain confidentiality described within these paragraphs exists both during the period that the search is active and to a reasonable time thereafter as determined by the chair. The retention of search records shall be in compliance with institutional and any applicable legal guidelines, and the disposition of records in a manner that retains candidate confidentiality.

6. Within 30 days of the conclusion of the work of the hiring committee, I will transfer all related files and all confidential information in my possession to the hiring committee chair for appropriate retention as part of the official records of the hiring committee.

I have read, understand, and agree to abide by all of the terms of this agreement as a condition of my service to the [organization] in its search for an empowerment evaluator.

_____

Signature

_____

Date

[15] Adapted from Ohio Domestic Violence Network

Appendix D: Sample Job Announcement[16]

Metropolitan Area Women's Center

Job Announcement

Job Title: Empowerment Evaluator

Type of Position: Part-time; contract position

Background:

The mission of the Metropolitan Area Women's Center (MAWC) is to eliminate domestic violence and sexual violence by changing societal attitudes, practices, and policies that support these types of violence through education, activism, advocacy, counseling, emergency shelter services, collaboration and partnerships. MAWC has received funding from the Alota Mulla Foundation to implement and evaluate a by-stander strategy for preventing intimate partner and sexual violence among teenagers.

Summary of Position:

The empowerment evaluation consultant will assist MAWC in building its organizational capacity to implement and evaluate a by-stander strategy for preventing intimate partner and sexual violence among teenagers. The empowerment evaluator will provide tools, training and technical assistance to MAWC staff and stakeholders in:

1. conducting a needs assessment to identify the area middle-school most appropriate to receive the by-stander strategy,

2. assessing the by-stander strategy's design to ensure that it is based on sound behavioral change principles and theory as well as compatible with the school's implementation context,

3. conducting a process evaluation, and

4. conducting an outcome evaluation,

The empowerment evaluator will also provide recommendations on how to increase organizational evaluation capacity throughout the term of the contract with MAWC. The empowerment evaluator will not be independently conducting an evaluation of the by-stander strategy, but supporting MAWC staff in improving their ability to implement and evaluate the by-stander strategy so that it is better able to achieve its stated goals and objectives.

Desired Qualifications:

- Minimum: M.A. degree in public health, psychology, social work, or related field.

- Preferred: Ph.D. degree in public health, psychology, social work, or related field.

- A minimum of 3 years (5 years preferred) of evaluation experience, preferably with specific experience working with organizations committed to ending violence against women and/or working with organizations focused on prevention,

- Course work in statistics and research methods and proficiency in using statistical database software.

- Knowledge of assessment techniques including survey, interview, observations, and focus groups.

- Excellent oral and written communication skills, with experience training adults.

- Congenial personality and ability to form strong working relationships with many diverse groups.

Job Responsibilities:

- Work from an empowerment evaluation framework.

- Travel to three trainings per year organized by the Alota Mulla Foundation, the funder of the by-stander program.

- Facilitate the development of an implementation plan for the by-stander strategy based on a needs assessment and assessment of the strategy's design by providing tools, training and technical assistance to MAWC staff members and key stakeholders,

- Facilitate the development of an evaluation plan for the by-stander strategy that includes both process and outcome evaluation activities by providing tools, training and technical assistance to MAWC staff members and key stakeholders,

- Coach MAWC staff members and key stakeholders as they implement and evaluate the by-stander strategy.

- Provide recommendations on how to increase organizational evaluation capacity throughout the term of the contract with MAWC.

How to Apply:

E-mail a letter of interest and your resume or vita to Jane Doe at [e-mail] by November 1, 2009. Call [phone] with questions.

[16] Adapted from samples used by various DELTA and EMPOWER Program grantees.

Appendix E:
Sample Request For Proposals[17]

Request for Proposal (RFP)
Anystate Department of Health

Funding available for an empowerment evaluator to join state intimate partner and sexual violence prevention team in supporting five local organizations in implementing and evaluating a by-stander strategy intended to prevent violence against women

A. Statement of Purpose

The Anystate Department of Health announces the availability of funds to hire an empowerment evaluator to work with the state intimate partner and sexual violence prevention team in supporting five local organizations in implementing and evaluating a by-stander strategy that is intended to prevent violence against women.

B. Background

The Anystate Department of Health has formed a partnership with the Anystate Coalition Against Sexual Assault, Anystate Coalition Against Domestic Violence, and the Governor's Advisory Council Against Domestic and Sexual Violence to address the issue of intimate partner and sexual violence prevention in Anystate. This partnership developed a statewide strategic plan that focuses on the primary prevention of intimate partner and sexual violence. One aspect of this plan calls for the implementation and evaluation of a by-stander strategy intended to prevent violence against women in five local communities. Five local organizations that address intimate partner and/or sexual violence have been selected to implement and evaluate the same by-stander strategy. The empowerment evaluator will be supporting these local organizations in their implementation and evaluation efforts related to this by-stander strategy. The evaluator will not be conducting an independent evaluation of the by-stander strategy. The empowerment evaluator will focus on building the evaluation capacity of the local organizations and their staff in:

1. conducting a needs assessment to identify the area middle-school most appropriate to receive the by-stander strategy,

2. assessing the by-stander strategy's design to ensure that it is based on sound behavioral change principles and theory as well as compatible with the school's implementation context,

3. conducting a process evaluation, and

4. conducting an outcome evaluation,

The empowerment evaluator will also provide recommendations on how to increase the organizational evaluation capacity of these five local organizations and how the state intimate partner and sexual violence prevention team can better support the evaluation efforts of these local organizations throughout the term of the contract.

C. Applicant Eligibility

- Minimum: M.A. degree in public health, psychology, evaluation, or related field.

- Preferred: Ph.D. degree in public health, psychology, evaluation, or related field.

- A minimum of 3 years (5 years preferred) of evaluation experience, preferably with specific experience working with domestic violence and sexual violence organizations, and/or working with organizations focused on prevention, and/or working with community coalitions and/or collaborative partnerships.

- Course work in statistics and research methods and proficiency in using statistical database software.

- Knowledge of assessment techniques including survey, interview, observations, and focus groups.

- Excellent oral and written communication skills, with experience training adults.

- Congenial personality and ability to form strong working relationships with many diverse groups.

D. Funding Information

Approximately $[amount] per year for 3 years for a part-time contract position. The 3-year funding and project period will begin in [month, year]. Travel, hotel, and per diem costs associated with required technical assistance trainings will be covered.

[17] Adapted from New Jersey Department of Community Affairs

E. Evaluator Responsibilities

- Work from an empowerment evaluation framework.

- Travel to three trainings per year organized by the Anystate Department of Health, the funder of the by-stander strategy.

- Facilitate the development of separate implementation plans for the by-stander strategy for each local organization based on a needs assessment and assessment of the strategy's design by providing tools, training and technical assistance to local organization staff members and key stakeholders,

- Facilitate the development of separate evaluation plans for the by-stander strategy for each local organization that includes both process and outcome evaluation activities by providing tools, training and technical assistance to local organization staff members and key stakeholders,

- Coach local organization staff members and key stakeholders as they implement and evaluate the by-stander strategy.

- Provide recommendations on how to increase organizational evaluation capacity of these five local organizations and how the state intimate partner and sexual violence prevention team can better support the evaluation efforts of these local organizations throughout the term of the contract.

F. Proposal Requirements

Describe how you will assist the state prevention team in supporting five local organizations in implementing and evaluating a by-stander strategy that is intended to prevent violence against women, paying special attention to how you will incorporate the 10 principles of empowerment evaluation into your tools, training and technical assistance. Include a proposed timeline and budget for the first year of project.

G. Review Process

1. Proposals received by the deadline will be reviewed by members of the intimate partner and sexual violence prevention team.

2. Interviews will be conducted the week of January 16, 2010.

3. Selection will be made by January 30, 2010.

H. Submission of Proposal

Interested individuals may e-mail or mail a letter of interest, proposal, and resume or vita to Mark Noname no later than 4:00PM, Friday, [month], [year].

E-mail:	[e-mail address]
Address:	[Name], Director of Public Education
	[State] Department of Health [Address]

For more information call [name] at [phone number].

Appendix F: Sample Interview Questions[18]

Questions About Evaluation Orientation and/or Empowerment Evaluation

- How would you describe your evaluation approach or orientation?

- What is your familiarity with empowerment evaluation? Have you ever done empowerment evaluation or participatory evaluation? If so, what were the challenges, successes, and lessons learned from your experience?

- This organization is looking for an evaluator who will assist in building organizational evaluation capacity through an approach called empowerment evaluation. Is this something you are willing and able to do?

- What does coaching an evaluation team within the organization mean to you? What are your expectations of the organization? What would be the first hint that this organization is not meeting your expectations regarding how empowerment evaluation should be done?

- How does empowerment evaluation compare with the way you normally work? What would you need to do differently to do empowerment evaluation?

- What is the fundamental difference between empowerment evaluation and other approaches to evaluation?

- Do you think process evaluation is important? Why or why not?

- Describe an example of how your evaluation findings were used to improve a strategy.

- What are your professional strengths as an empowerment evaluator? What are your professional challenges?

Questions Related to Fees

What is your fee structure or schedule? Is it negotiable? If so, what parts (i.e., indirect rate or hourly rate)?

- Do you prefer a fixed-fee contract or a time and materials contract?

- How do you normally get reimbursed for travel? Do you charge for travel time? Do you have a minimum daily per diem?

Questions Related to the Position Being Offered

- When you read the job description for this position, what appealed to you most about the position?

- If offered this position, what challenges do you expect to face?

- What previous work experience do you have as an evaluator that is particularly relevant or similar to the position this organization has available?

- Are you able to devote the necessary hours per week or days per month for this project?

- Are you able and willing to travel for this position?

Questions about Cultural Competence

- Describe your experiences working with culturally and racially diverse groups.

- What is your definition of **cultural competence?** How does your definition go beyond language translation?

- Describe cross-cultural communication models or techniques to collaborate with communities to understand and address their needs through evaluation.

- What are some barriers you've experienced in integrating diversity issues into evaluation? How have you addressed them?

- What measures would you take to minimize or eliminate marginalization through the evaluation process?

- How do you promote cultural competence in your work, even when it may limit the rigor of the evaluation process?

[18] Developed and used by various DELTA and EMPOWER Program grantees.

Questions About Negotiating Challenges, Facilitating Collaboration, and Building Capacity Among Community Groups

- How would you promote stakeholder buy-in of empowerment evaluation on this project?

- What experience do you have training adults? Providing technical assistance to adults?

- Hypothetical scenario: You've met with all the local community groups a few times now, and you have noticed that at one site in particular, there is a lack of investment in the evaluation process. Several key team members have been absent from meetings and during the meetings, participants are often distracted with other crises, or they seem anxious and preoccupied with completing the required reports and paperwork for the evaluation, and show little interest in the process for genuine reflection and learning. What would you do in this situation?

- Hypothetical scenario: While working with the statewide steering committee at their regular meeting, it becomes clear that two members are challenging the chairs and the group and promoting philosophical conflict about use of gender-based issues. How would approach this situation?

Questions When Interviewing an Evaluation Team (Firms/ Organizations or University-Based)

- Briefly describe the history, mission, and focus of your organization/firm. Please highlight a couple of relevant accomplishments.

- Describe your team structure. How is work distributed? Is there a team leader?

- Describe the experience and background of each person on the team.

- How much time is each person on your team available to work on the project (hours per week)? Will availability change over time?

- What about this contract do you think would challenge you or your organization or team? What strengths does your team possess that would help you manage the contract?

- How does your organization or team prioritize work among competing projects? Will team members be working on multiple projects?

- Will graduate students be involved in the project? How will they be selected? Will they be involved throughout the whole project or come and go based on semester/course requirements?

- How will graduate students be supervised? Who will monitor the quality and timeliness of their work? Will they be paid?

- Give us some examples of how your team would cope with shifts in priority among projects. For example, if you have five requests for technical assistance in one week, how would your team prioritize needs and feasibility of response?

- Describe the management structure for ensuring that deliverables are submitted on time and of sufficient quality.

Appendix G: Sample Budget and Narrative for an Evaluation Team[19]

Year 1 Budget

	Percentage of Time Devoted to Project	Budget
Personnel		
Salary and Wages—Faculty		
Project Coordinator	10%	$4,488
Evaluation Analyst	20%	$9,117
Evaluation Assistant	50%	$26,330
Admin. Support	8%	$2,897
Business Office Support	5%	$2,015
Total Salary		$44,847
Fringe Benefits (35%) – see narrative for description		$15,696
Total Salary & Fringe Benefits		**$60,543**
Operating		
Travel		$7,650
in-state: 21 trips, 1 person	$4,784	
in-state: 3 trips to Capital City x 4 people	$1,866	
evaluation training conference, 1 person	$1,000	
Communications		$420
postage, telecommunications	$420	
Office Supplies		$1,425
duplicating, printing, supplies including	$300	
50 evaluation binders @ $22.50 ea	$1,125	
Other		$1,710
annual evaluation workshop	$1,710	
Total Operating		**$11,205**
Subtotal		**$71,748**
Indirect Rate (9%)		$6,457
Total Costs Requested		**$78,205**

[19] Adapted from the North Dakota Council on Abused Women's Services/Coalitions Against Sexual Assault.

Budget Justification

A. Personnel

Funds in the amount of $44,847 are requested to support University of Our State (UOS) salaries as listed below. Funds in the amount of $15,696 are requested to support fringe benefits. Fringe benefits are based on historical data and estimated at 35 percent for faculty and staff; the actual cost of benefits will be charged to the grant.

Project Coordinator will provide overall leadership and guidance for the project including overseeing the implementation of all project-related activity. She will act as the lead on conference calls and meetings with partner organizations and at training events. She will be responsible for disseminating all written products at the conclusion of the project. She will provide 10% effort to the project.

Evaluation Analyst will implement the empowerment evaluation component of the project, overseeing all other team member's evaluation activities. He will provide in-house training to colleagues as needed and act as the lead analyst. He will participate in team meetings and conference calls and attend evaluator trainings. He will provide 20% effort to the project.

Evaluation Assistant will implement the empowerment evaluation model with assigned communities. This position will assist with the overall project as needed, including attendance at meetings, travel to communities, workshop training, and tracking efforts. This position will be filled by the start of the project and will provide 70% effort to the project.

Administrative Support will provide support services to the project including scheduling of meetings and conference calls, travel arrangements, document production, duplication of project materials, dissemination of information, and other project-specific tasks as assigned. Administrative support, garnered from current UOS staff, will provide 8% effort to the project.

Business Office Support will monitor the budget and process reimbursement requests as needed. Business office support, garnered from current UOS staff, will provide 5% effort to the project.

Fringe Benefits include life insurance 3%, OASDI (Social Security) 7%, Medicare 3%, unemployment insurance 3%, health care insurance14%, and 401(k) contribution 5%.

B. Equipment

Not anticipated.

C. Travel

Funds in the amount of $4,784 are requested for three site visits travel to each of the 21 grantee locations (1 person). Funds in the amount of $1,866 are requested for travel to Capital City for four people to attend three statewide trainings for grantees. Additional travel funding in the amount of $1,000 is requested for an evaluation team member to attend evaluation training projected to be held in Capital City.

D. Communications

Funds in the amount of $420 are requested for postage and telecommunication costs.

E. Supplies

Funds in the amount of $1,425 are requested for project-specific supplies. This includes paper, toner, and other necessary small desk supplies as well as the cost of duplication, which will consist primarily of grantee binders including evaluation materials.

F. Other Costs

Funds in the amount of $1,710 are requested for other costs, including those associated with statewide training including meeting room, breaks, lunch, and speaker fees.

G. Total Direct Costs

$71,747

H. Indirect Costs

UOS's federally approved indirect cost rate for non-research projects is 30%. The funding organization limits indirect costs to 9%. Funds in the amount of $6,457 are requested for indirect costs.

This project will have access to video and audio teleconferencing, computer support services, educational technology support, multi-media presentation technology including web casting, medical library support, and electronic document management available to all projects based in the University of Our State. UOS supports this project by providing the necessary administrative structure (payroll, accounting services) as well as access to campus services (libraries, labs, meeting rooms). This project will be afforded full availability of the above-mentioned resources, as needed to achieve the objectives of this grant.

I. Total Funds Requested

$78,204

Evaluation for Improvement = Empowerment Evaluation